Time, Health and Medicine

Time, Health and Medicine

edited by

Ronald Frankenberg

SAGE Publications
London • Newbury Park • New Delhi

Chapter 1 © Ronald Frankenberg
Chapter 2 © Cecil Helman
Chapter 3 © Hilary Thomas
Chapter 4 © Franca Pizzini
Chapter 5 © Peter Pritchard
Chapter 6 © Ken Starkey
Chapter 7 © Paul Bellaby
Chapter 8 © Alan Prout
Chapter 9 © Pat Allatt
Chapter 10 © Barbara Adam

First published 1992

 SAGE Publications Ltd
6 Bonhill Street
London EC2A 4PU

SAGE Publications Inc
2455 Teller Road
Newbury Park, California 91320

SAGE Publications India Pvt Ltd
32, M-Block Market
Greater Kailash – I
New Delhi 110 048

British Library Cataloguing in Publication Data
Time, Health and Medicine
  I. Frankenberg, Ronald
306.4

ISBN 0-8039-8678-5

Library of Congress catalog card number 91-051133

Typeset by GCS, Leighton Buzzard, Bedfordshire
Printed in Great Britain by Billing & Sons Ltd, Worcester

Contents

Preface

The papers here collected are not a random assemblage but constitute the product of, and reflect, the shared and overlapping pasts of their writers. They are presented to incorporate not only a vision of these authors' future concerns but as a hopeful invitation to others to join or rejoin the discussion of health, healing, medicine and time with a critical focus on the last. No sense of closure or finality is intended or achieved. Indeed Barbara Adam's concluding paper here correctly and sharply draws attention to the general absence of, and pressing need for, a focus on the working out of the dialectic within health of internally and externally derived personal body time. At various times Pat Allatt, Paul Bellaby, Ronnie Frankenberg and Alan Prout have worked together on problems of the sociology of health and illness at Keele. Their work converged with Hilary Thomas's at Cambridge through meetings of both the British Sociological Association's Medical Sociology Group and of ASSET where they renewed their own commitment and, encouraged by Michael Young and Tom Schuller, met and joined forces with Barbara Adam, Peter Pritchard and Ken Starkey. I must personally acknowledge a great, continuing but not yet totally assimilated, influence of phenomenologically-oriented US, British and European social and cultural anthropologists (see Gaines and Hahn, 1985; Frankenberg, 1988; Lock and Gordon, 1988; Csordas, 1990) although this volume is concerned almost entirely with time and health in a Western industrial context. Franca Pizzini, part of similar processes in Italy, has been persuaded to join her writings to ours since, although invited, she was not able to attend either the ASSET or the Royal Anthropological Institute conferences where some of the papers were first presented. Cecil Helman gave a preliminary version of the paper reprinted here at the latter. Barbara Adam has read and commented fruitfully on all the papers at an earlier stage in the book's preparation.

Each paper, of course, can stand and be read meaningfully on its own or in association with the author's other works. I have reprinted my own 'Your Time and Mine' as an introduction to the way that in the practice of biomedicine, boundaries of time, like those of space and the body, are inevitably fortified and emphasized while being breached. It is, I suggest, from these tragic and unavoidable contradictions that medicine derives its strengths and its weaknesses, its popularity and its unpopularity. We love our physicians because they share our time with us; we hate them because they incorporate it into their own. Helman's paper (Chapter 2) reinforces this general approach in his striking demonstration of the way that the cultures of heart disease and of Western industrial society mutually influence and even create one another. After these introductory papers, the others are arranged as a kind of collage/narrative starting within the boundaries of the mindful body (Scheper Hughes and Lock, 1987) in Hilary Thomas's paper (Chapter 3) on time and the cervix uteri. In the next (Chapter 4) Franca Pizzini discusses the increasing contradiction of body time and the dominance of calendar and clock time during and after birth in a Milan maternity hospital. Then Peter Pritchard (Chapter 5) moves us back once more into the practitioner's surgery where the secular (ie, cut off) time-management exigencies of clock and calendar come most sharply into conflict with the patients' perception of their own body time as continuous unsegmented flow. Ken Starkey (Chapter 6) moves still further into doctors' territory in the world of the hospital and is even able to discuss consultant physicians' time with, as his problem seems to allow, little reference to that of patients' at all. He opens the door for our understanding, in the papers of Paul Bellaby (Chapter 7) and Alan Prout (Chapter 8), of the social, cultural (and political economical) construction of time in two other work places those of the adult-factory, and of the child-school. In these sites the mindful body seems almost totally subservient to the time definitions of the bodies social and politic. Penultimately, with a neat reversal of causation, Pat Allatt (Chapter 9) shows how for the unemployed and their relatives, disorders of time are perceived as disorders of the body and are so metaphorically described by those who suffer them, opening the way to Barbara Adam's salutary and indeed timely reflections not only on the effects of scholarly and lay perceptions and analysis of conventional boundaries, but also on the very existence of meaningful boundaries at all between nature and culture, individual and society (Chapter 10).

The book is in fact focused on health in the context of exclusively Western medicine and it is fascinating to remind oneself how overtly and latently essential to that discourse are time concepts. Thus diseases are classified as acute and chronic; pandemic, epidemic and endemic according to how long they last and whether they are present everywhere at once, in many people at the same time and the same place, or always. The distinction made by many anthropologists and most sociologists between illness, disease and sickness also contains sharp time differentiations. Thus illness is perceived by the sufferer as part of a flow of trying or testing experiences (Michael Taussig, 1980; Barbara

Adam, 1989) which has become salient or dominant at a point of time. If, impatient of suffering, the pre-patient singles illness out for legitimation and diagnosis, it becomes a disease recognized by a physician. This has an episodic quality, a sanctioned beginning and an end, often recognized in law as well as in medicine. It is necessary in medical theory to find the point of onset of disease and to know its likely duration with or without interventions. Furthermore, notwithstanding the writings of historians like Figlio (1982), sociologists like Gabbay (1982) and anthropologists like Lewis (1987), disease concepts themselves are seen as timeless and unchanging: asthma in the seventeenth century and today, leprosy at the time of Leviticus and in New Guinea are assumed to be the same. Finally, all the papers focus on sickness as *specific* cultural performance which conceptually as in real life is always situated in an equally specific historic space and time.

References

Adam, B. (1989) 'Feminist Social Theory Needs Time', *Sociological Review*, 37(3): 458–73.

Csordas, T.S. (1990) 'Embodiment as a Paradigm for Anthropology', *Ethos*, 18: 5–47.

Figlio, K. (1982) 'How does Illness Mediate Social Relations: Workmen's Compensation and Medico-Legal Practices 1899–1940', in P. Wright and A. Treacher (eds), *The Problem of Medical Knowledge: Examining the Social Construction of Medicine*. Edinburgh: Edinburgh University Press. pp. 174–224.

Frankenberg, R. (1988) ' "Your Time or Mine?" An Anthropological View of the Tragic Temporal Contradictions of Biomedical Practice', *International Journal of Health Services*, 18: 111–34.

Gabbay, J. (1982) 'Asthma Attacked? Tactics for the Reconstruction of a Disease Concept', in P. Wright and A. Treacher (eds), *The Problem of Medical Knowledge: Examining the Social Construction of Medicine*. Edinburgh: Edinburgh University Press. pp. 23–48.

Gaines, A.D. and Hahn, R.A. (1985) *Physicians of Western Medicine: Anthropological Approaches to Theory and Practice*. Dordrecht: Kluwer. pp. ix and 345.

Helman, C. (1987) 'Heart Disease and the Cultural Construction of Time: The Type A Behaviour Pattern as a Western Culture Bound Syndrome', *Social Science and Medicine*, 25(9): 69–79.

Lewis, G. (1987) 'A Lesson from Leviticus: Leprosy', *Man*, 22(4): 593–612.

Lock, M. and Gordon, D. (eds) (1988) *Biomedicine Examined*. Dordrecht: Kluwer. pp. vii and 558.

Scheper Hughes, N. and Lock, M. (1987) 'The Mindful Body: A Prolegomenon to Future Work in Medical Anthropology', *Medical Anthropology Quarterly*, NS1: 16–41.

Taussig, M. (1980) 'Reification and the Consciousness of the Patient', *Social Science and Medicine*, 14: 3–13.

Notes on Contributors

Barbara Adam received her PhD from the University of Wales and is currently Lecturer in Social Theory at the University of Wales College of Cardiff. She is editor of *Time and Society* and has written numerous articles on social time. Her book *Time and Social Theory* won the Philip Abrams Memorial Prize awarded by the British Sociological Association for best first book.

Pat Allatt is Reader at Teesside Business School. She has researched and published on burglary, the youth service, youth labour markets, women, social policy and the family, and is currently engaged in ESRC 16–19 Initiative, researching the development of young people's economic and political identities within the family household.

Paul Bellaby is Senior Lecturer in Sociology and Director of the Centre for Health Policy Research at the University of East Anglia, Norwich. His publications cover the comprehensive school, the organization of nursing and social work, occupational health, risk behaviour and accidents and the life course.

Ronald Frankenberg is Professor Emeritus of Sociology and Social Anthropology at the University of Keele where he now teaches a Master's programme as Professorial Research Fellow and Director of the Centre for Medical Social Anthropology. He is also Professor Associate in the Centre for the Study of Health Sickness and Disablement and teaches on the M.Sc programme in Medical Anthropology at Brunel University in West London. His writings include *Village on the Border* (1957 and 1989) *Communities in Britain* 1966, and the edited volume *Custom and Conflict in British Society* 1982. He has worked on health care in Lusaka, Zambia and in Italy. His current research interests are AIDS/HIV, the cultural performance of sickness, temporality in Biomedicine, and narratives of chronic suffering.

Cecil Helman is Professor Associate of Medical Anthropology at Brunel University, Senior Lecturer in Primary Health Care at University College and Middlesex Medical School, and Research Fellow in Anthropology, University College London. He is particularly interested in psychosomatic and culture-bound disorders. He is the author of the textbook *Culture, Health and Illness: An Introduction for Health Professionals* (1990).

Franca Pizzini is tenured Research Fellow at the Department of Sociology, University of Milan. For many years she has done research on human reproductive issues, with particular attention to the women's point of view. She has published books and articles in Italian and English and is currently working on a book called *Reproductive Technologies*.

Peter Pritchard has been a general practitioner in Oxfordshire since 1951. He is a former part-time lecturer in the Department of Social and Administrative Studies at University of Oxford and Ruskin College; and a former member of the Oxford Regional Health Authority. He is currently senior medical adviser to the Advanced Computation Laboratory of the Imperial Cancer Research Fund.

Alan Prout is Lecturer at the Department of Sociology and Social Anthropology at the University of Keele, and Course Director at the Centre for Medical Social Anthropology. He was previously Senior Lecturer at South Bank Polytechnic and Senior Research Associate at the Child Care and Development Group, University of Cambridge.

Ken Starkey is Reader in Organizational Analysis in the School of Management and Finance, University of Nottingham. His interests cover the management of time, particularly among professional groups and the general areas of strategic management and organizational analysis.

Hilary Thomas is Lecturer in Medical Sociology in the Department of Sociology, University of Surrey, and at Frances Harrison College of Healthcare. Her particular interests are in women's health, and narratives of time and the body.

1

'Your Time or Mine': temporal contradictions of biomedical practice

Ronald Frankenberg

It does not require a very introspective patient to see the surface connection between time and his or her experience of medicine. Medicine seems, at least in its present manifestation (Armstrong, 1984, 1985), like some of those described by the culture and personality school, to be a waiting culture. Surgeries or physicians' offices usually have a waiting room and one waits to see the doctor a matter of minutes and hours, for treatments a matter of days or weeks, and for 'cold' surgical operations a matter of months or years. Indeed, a pharmacist employed by a major English drugstore chain testified to a Nuffield Foundation enquiry that, while it was possible to dispense some medicines in a matter of seconds by reaching up and taking a package from the shelf, it was company policy to impose a delay so that patients would realize as a result of having to wait that drugs were not just commodities (and he might have added that pharmacists were professionals and not mere shop assistants) (Nuffield Foundation, 1986).

For physicians, and other health workers as well, time is not peripheral but of the essence. Physicans have first of all the longest period of training of any professional (save the veterinary surgeon) and during that training work longer and more irregular hours than any fellow students. They have the shortest vacations and during post-graduate training their time is literally not their own. The notoriously and (in terms of patient care) irrationally long hours of what in the United Kingdom are called junior hospital doctors and in the United States interns can be seen as a symbolic initiation into their opposite, the sacred, inviolable time of the qualified physician, which is protected and parcelled out by his or her supporters. (But see the paradox of the breach of sacred norms below, p. 5.) There is the same asymmetry between the value of the consulting patients' time and that of their doctors as there is between the sovereign's or the president's and that of their attendant ministers and press corps, and largely for the same reasons, both functional and symbolic. The principal actor in the performance is a scarce, even unique, good and has symbolic value above and beyond his or her scarcity value. Thus, at least in the 1950s, ministers of the crown were required by court officials to attend at Buckingham Palace 30 minutes before the time of an audience, while the Queen, showing the politeness of princes, appeared always exactly on the appointed hour. Relative status was thus doubly enforced. Senior doctors and other worthies attending meetings of the (British) General Medical Council arrive ten minutes or so in advance and proceed into the council chamber punctually together, sensitively avoiding the exercise of that time power over their peers to which they routinely subject their patients (Stacey and Prendergast, 1986).

Thus in Robert A. Hahn's fascinating but disturbing in-depth description of an internist (to English readers something between a general practitioner with hospital rights and a consultant physician) whom he calls Barry Siegler, he writes:

> Barry's life is scheduled far in advance. He knows when he will take his vacation next year, which weekends and nights he is 'on call,' which mornings he will make rounds in which hospital, and the hourly contours of each day. These plans are generally changed only for emergencies – those of patients, colleagues, and his family. Patient emergencies are the business of being on call, but these and other emergencies may also interrupt the remainder of the schedule as well.
>
> Barry's time is structured by degrees of medical engagement – of access by patients, and of his reciprocal obligation to respond. Each partner has intense time 'on,' but certain time 'off' as well. Each is 'covered' by his partners when he is 'off.' These states significantly define the physician's role. Barry once referred to periods spent in the hospital as 'clump time' and to periods at home waiting to be called as 'scattered time.' While in the hospital, medical work is continuous; call at home leaves him continuously susceptible to medical interruption. Emergency call reaches the office [*Anglice*, surgery] as well. When I first went to meet Barry in his office, to explain my study and to ask to accompany him, he had left the office without warning to go to the hospital where his patient was admitted with an 'MI' (myocardial infarction or heart attack). I left to return another time; scheduled patients were delayed.
>
> Barry's schedule marks out his location and the general scope of his work there at different times, but not which patients he will see or what specific problems he will have to treat. The schedule provides slots for work whose size is limited in several dimensions. Certain problems can be dealt with in the hospital, but not in the office, or in the afternoon hospital working visits, but not in hospital rounds, or in the intensive care unit, but not 'on the floor,' and so on. Barry tries to fit the work into his schedule. If parts do not fit, they are abandoned or postponed, or the schedule expands, extending, Barry's day, deferring and reordering other appointments. He 'runs behind.'
>
> Barry is oppressed by two sorts of temporal constraints: too much to do in the allotted time, and the urgency of action imposed by what are too often literal 'deadlines.' Time is differently shaped accordingly: excess draws it out, imminence intensifies each moment.

Barry's day begins with rounds, sometimes at one, sometimes at the other of two (out of town) Cartown hospitals to which he and his partners admit patients. He is accompanied by the residents and sometimes by medical students on his service. The rounds run from 7:30 to 9:00 am or shortly after 9:00 am, when Barry goes to the group office, several miles away. He has breakfast in the hospital, often with the residents and students (and during the period of this study, an anthropologist) and in one of the hospitals with an obstetrician friend or another physician. Talk at breakfast is often about recent recreational activity, sports events or food. Sometimes, Barry will be in the hospital before breakfast, to read his patients' electrocardiograms and other laboratory reports. (Hahn, 1985: 61–2)

Despite the gruelling schedule, in this case, shared for the five months of the study by one of those academics whom Barry normally despises as having too much time on their hands (ibid.: 78), the symbolic asymmetry with patients other than the actually dying remains:

Barry always tries to leave the hospital for the office around 9:00 am, so that he does not make office patients wait. He rushes to leave, impatient; he often postpones until the afternoon what he planned or hoped to do in the morning. Still, he notes, patients sometimes wait as long as two hours to see him. Most patients are scheduled far in advance; others 'squeeze-ins,' call with problems felt to be urgent, and are seen if the partners and/or staff concur on the urgency. I suspect that except in the most extraordinary of circumstances, perhaps a serious plea from a valued community colleague, only Barry's or his partners' own patients would have this immediate access to his attention. Barry says that he himself waits about five minutes every five years, when patients do not show up. (ibid.: 69–70)

It is clear that the expenditure of time, like shifts in space – home, office (or, in the United Kingdom, surgery), hospital – has important symbolic value in the ambiance of medicine and healing, what I choose to call the cultural performance of sickness. This, of course, has not hitherto passed unnoticed, whether by the patients who suffer and perhaps thereby earn their cure through it, by the consultants who manipulate and enhance their status through it, or by sociologists such as Zerubavel (1979) who have recorded it and thereby received their doctorates. Turner (1985: 227–46), in a paper first published in 1981, introduces a concept of 'anti-temporality' to analyse the immunity from sanctions of an irreverent, treasonable, and satirical clown within a South Indian temple ceremony. In those circumstances, his performance was seen by those present as taking place in 'timeless time'. One can contrast such absolute anti-temporality with the relative anti-temporality that distinguishes the hospital from the world outside. Time inside is real enough as is time outside. Each, however, has its own idiom independent of the other but transformable by the ceremonies of admission for patients, donning white coats and name tags for the staff. Thus the preoperation abstentions are only regarded as reliable if the patient spent the previous night in hospital; the apparently healthy are moved from front door to ward by wheelchair, and impertinent penetrations into the body physical are made as pertinent as the holy clown's penetration into the body social, not by necessity, but by translation into a new world of time.[1]

In this chapter, I seek to analyse the reality with a greater emphasis on the study of the culture, in addition to the organization, of health and sickness and their associated institutions.

A classical medical sociological approach

From novels and personal reminiscences as well as such sociological studies as Julius Roth's *Timetables* (1963) or Zerubavel's *Patterns of Time in Hospital Life* (1979) we can see that for the patients, the passage of time in hospital appears to continue inflexibly from routine with almost total disruption of the 'normal, natural' rhythms of bodily desires: to sleep or to go on sleeping, to eat or to refrain from eating, to evacuate waste solids and liquids, and to enjoy sexual experience. Indeed, as the nature of jokes in hospital films and television series shows, no time or space at all is legitimately allowed for the latter. (For a poignant and suitably sanctioned exception see Collier and Horowitz, 1985: 594.) A whole genre of comedy is based on these disruptions, both iatrogenic and bureaucratic, of the temporal basis of motions across body boundaries. Even in 'Hospital Romances' it is only significant glances that are exchanged in hospital time. Penetrations of the mildest osculatory kind take place in off-duty times and places.

The time experience of both doctors and nurses is not only markedly different from that of patients but is also itself quite diverse. For nurses there is a scheduling of time even more rigorous than that for the patients since it is both externally sanctioned and ingrained. Within a variation imposed by the exigencies of a system of shifts, nurses come to work at fixed times and proceed through a liminal period of changeover, to a fixed-period shift. When the shift ends, whatever crisis may be in train, it ends definitively for all nurses of that shift. They go off duty for a determined, bounded period of rest and do not, in any circumstances, return until they are next on duty. In Strauss et al.'s (1985) terms, sentimental work may be an essential part of the nurse's duties for the dying and for the giving birth but the sentimental worker like other workers is not merely substitutable but has substitution imposed upon him or her by clock-regulated schedules. For nurses then, private time and public time are clearly demarcated, and so thereby is their use of the public space of the ward and their role in the lives of their patients. In US hospitals, nurses' work-time is measured and paid for by the hour (Zerubavel, 1979: 16). The continuous vigil at the bedside is reserved for kin: parents of immature sick children, husbands of those in labour, expectant widows, and the mature children of sick and dying parents.

The yearly-paid doctors, of course, also have their fixed points: ward rounds, clinics, and fixed times for particular procedures when it is necessary that patient, nurse, technician, porter, and physician or surgeon should all be in the same place at the same time.[2] However, there is no time of day or night when the expectation of their presence is unthinkable or when they cannot, at least in theory, be summoned. Nor is the appearance of a doctor on the ward at any time, whether or not he or she is known to be on duty, in principle the matter of remark or speculation. The ultimate sign or perhaps even symbol of this is the bleep (in the United States, beeper), which has supplemented the label, the white coat, and the stethoscope. While the latter emphasize the incumbency of a role in space and at a particular time, the bleep implies that the persona and the individual are never separated for long even in sleep, at meals, in the washroom, or the erotic embrace. The boundaries of private and public space and time are, again in theory, as totally disrupted as they are for the inmate of the total institution. But whereas in the latter context this marks a loss of status, for the hospital doctor it is a symbol of almost sacred power and powers. For him or her there is not only no boundary between private and public, but also none between night and day and hence by extension between death and life. The fact that night time as a 'frontier' (Giddens, 1984: 119) is so marked in the hospital, as every patient knows, serves to emphasize still further the mystery of those who cross it so easily. This, of course, is only fitting for those licensed in the course of duty to cross, even to penetrate, the boundaries between the embodied self and the self-in-the-world.

Zerubavel's conclusion that the flexibility of time scheduling is inversely related to status and power within the hospital, while it stimulated this analysis, is perhaps too simple to encompass the symbolic realities involved. Just as St Francis and his followers derive their holy powers (and my use of the plural is deliberate) not from being poor but from their choice of poverty, so senior doctors (for example, in the United Kingdom, consultants) derive theirs from the choice of forgoing the privilege of private time. The choice is not available to nurses and their status is diminished because they are denied it. The time status of hospital midwives, not specially summoned back to duty but allowed to remain to see a birth through, provides an interesting limiting and intermediate case.

While it seems to be the case that natural rhythms decree that deaths, disease crises, and births most often occur at night, this also has social and cultural implications. It may be that the revolt of women against inductions and Caesarean births was made possible precisely by the fact that shifting birth to the daytime in these ways disrupted the symmetry of the equation: I have violated the boundaries between the physician's public and private time, she or he may violate the boundaries of my body self. It now became apparent that the obstetrician was exercising power instead of powers and his or her authority became literally and metaphorically questionable. Those physicians who wish to abdicate the responsibility thrust upon them to turn off life support machines should ensure that the operation is carried out between nine and five. Italian primary care physicians who work similar office hours have similarly deprived themselves of both mystery and status, which the Guardia Medica, who take their place at night, at the weekend, and on public holidays, do not gain since they are known not to be volunteers but pressed men (and women) compelled like any other night-shift worker by economic or family necessity.

Opposing approaches to medical anthropology

Arthur Kleinmau in his seminal and important works, which have done much to establish the bona fide nature of the subject among US physicians and especially psychiatrists, makes a distinction between disease and illness. He transfers to the study of 'illth'[3] in Western society a distinction spelled out and analysed in, for example, societies such as the Gnau in New Guinea, by writers such as Gilbert Lewis (1975: 148–9). Kleinman is able for the most part, by dividing illness and disease, to reassure his fellow physicians that their concepts of disease do not have to be rejected, their training is sound, and their understanding of pathological entities good. However, to be at their most effective in relation to curing or succouring their patients, they need the understanding of the meaning of disease to the sufferer that the study by medical anthropologists can illuminate, analyse, and in the most favourable circumstances, explain. This he calls illness (Kleinman, 1978, 1986). Medical care then, again in Strauss's general terminology of arcs of work (Strauss et al., 1985), involves educational work. The physician must learn the patient's interpretation and the nature of the illness, and then in turn, as part of the cure, teach the patient as much about the disease as is possible and necessary for treatment to be both carried out and complied with.

While such an approach certainly presents a conceptual advance and has led to other such advances as well as much valuable empirical work, I have in several earlier publications argued my feelings about its limitations. The approach seems to me to beg questions about the nature of healing by privileging unduly both the physician's definition of the nature of the illth and his or her role in bringing about cure or providing care. In this chapter, I hope by introducing ideas related to time to carry this criticism further. I feel this particularly apposite because in the context of academic study such an approach also tends, in my view, to make it more difficult to apply to Western medicine that kind of critical sociological attention that we give to systems that are less readily acceptable to Western scholars. At the same time it may, therefore, weaken our study of the latter. I have in mind an analogy with the strong programme in the sociology of science which holds that the sociological explanation for the acceptance of mathematics should not differ in kind from that needed to explain the acceptance of phrenology or ectoplasmic spiritualist manifestations (Bloor, 1976; Law and Lodge, 1984).

My own preferred conceptualization (Frankenberg and Leeson, 1976), derived originally from Suchman, but also having emic roots in the English language, is to add to Kleinman's disease and illness a concept of sickness that refers to the way that illth is socially and culturally performed.[4] Paying attention to sickness as cultural performance involves the scholar in a fruitful questioning of a set of interactions. In the Western case, relationships will be revealed between individuals and things, which include physicians, other health workers, sufferers, relatives, and friends as well as diverse objects with both instrumental and expressive functions in the total performance.

By disease, I mean a disturbance of body functions and performance seen in biological terms of the kind that physicians are primarily trained to detect, diagnose, and treat. Biology is also concerned with time both as the background to the evolution of life and its forms and, in smaller units, as a measure of the processes of morbidity and mortality. A disease, of course, can be seen in such terms as a temporary but potentially permanent interruption to the process that I have elsewhere called lifedeath in order to emphasize its finitude (Frankenberg, 1987), or as a speeding up or slowing down of life processes, or as a cutting short of lifedeath itself. However, as Gabbay (1982) has cogently pointed out, it is a common illusion of biomedicine to assume that part of the definition of diseases as diseases is their timelessness or perduring nature, whereas, as he has shown for asthma, its legitimate definition even at one point of time is hotly disputed within and between treatises.

Illness is concerned with the conceptions of sufferers of that which physicians conceive of as disease. Sufferers may observe themselves as being unable to achieve against a measurement of time what they could achieve before their illness. The meaning of segments of time may be disrupted or destroyed. It is still 8 o'clock but no longer time for breakfast, and times for play and for work may no longer have that subjective meaning. Enhanced consciousness of mortality may change time-meaning even more fundamentally. Again, as Zola (1972) pointed out, neither patients nor their friends, relatives, or doctors hesitate to move the onset of their illness back in time beyond the incidence of their disease. They recall staying out in the rain; not wearing warm clothes; not being careful where they trod; eating, drinking, and smoking inappropriately; and in general neglecting to keep themselves healthy. Murcott (1981) has described how clinical oncologists categorize and blame patients as 'bad' who are alleged to have delayed in reporting their symptoms. Both patients and, in many circumstances, doctors thereby date the origins of, and by implication responsibility for, their misfortunes in their own past misdemeanours. It may be that, for this and other reasons, in addition to distinguishing the best of bees from the worst of architects by their differential ability to plan the future, Marx would have been wise to compare also their capacities to reconstruct the past.

To me sickness is the key concept since it provides the social and cultural framework for the anthropologist to analyse the social consequences of illness and disease that are in this sense secondary. Disease depends on the existence of the social organization of biologists and the medically trained, and illness on a socially constructed sense of self, which certainly does not exist in the same form in all societies. Sickness as cultural performance can be analysed in all societies even if a specific performance may be the denial of disease and the absence of illness.[5]

The performance of sickness is always culturally specific, not only to particular times and places but also in relation to conditions of disease occurrence, such as epidemic, endemic, or individual. This is particularly clear among the Gnau, for example. They have a spirit, Taklei, who causes epidemics (Lewis, 1975: 81–2; 168–9); they do not bother to explain endemic diseases and they account for individual sickness in a large number of different ways, which Lewis shows are related to spirits of various kinds, to sorcery and magic, or to breaking of taboos. Actual cases in each category are explained by past events related to time sequences, places, the ingestion of food, and particular actions. Sickness among the Gnau as in all other societies always involves, by definition, a usage of time and space different from a situation where sickness is not performed. Cultural performance of sickness may or may not be influenced by changing views on the aetiology of disease (Gabbay, 1982: 26); it is certainly and always revealing about social relations in general since it is concerned with the management of the body and its boundaries, with the relationship of society to nature (Comaroff, 1982: 51), and with mortality and the transitions lifedeath, deathlife, and death.[6]

Just as in the case of illness, the cultural performance of sickness, like other performance, may require more or less systematic, notional reconstruction, through selective inattentions, of past actions through which present and future performance can be understood (Lewis, 1975: 227–8). There is an analogy with the theatre, where we usually meet characters fully mature and rely on their dialogue and nonverbal signs to deduce a past and a future in this case even more fictitious than their present. Roth has a striking example in his study of tuberculosis hospitals:

> [W]hen a medical resident presented a patient as having been in the hospital for two years, a consultant promptly announced: 'That's a long time; I think we should try and get her out of here.' One of the nurses pointed out that the resident had made a slight mistake on the matter of length of hospitalisation. The patient had first been admitted about two years ago, but had been discharged after about a year, had spent half a year on the outside, and had then been readmitted. Her second admission had involved slightly less than a six months' stay in the hospital. The consultant replied; 'I'd hate to let her go too soon this time.' This doctor then argued in favor of holding the patient for at least another conference six months later. All this time the physician was looking at exactly the same set of X-rays and was considering the same information concerning bacteriological tests and other diagnostic procedures. The only reason for the different position he took in his second statement was knowing that the patient had been out of hospital for a period of time and that her present period of hospitalization had been for only a relatively short time – obviously *too* short a time, in the doctor's opinion. (Roth, 1963: 28)

The cultural performance of sickness is an episode in not one but several time sequences for each of the performers. For a surgeon, a tonsillectomy may be merely the first of the day or the first of his or her career, but it is or is expected to be part of series of repetitive events that make up the surgeon's week, year, career, and life. For the patient it may mean a week removed from his or her life course and one that has been subjected to insertion in a different framework of time and space. For patients with burns or recurrent cancer or for leukaemic children (Bluebond-Langner, 1978) certain performances may be as familiar in a different way and as repetitive as for the surgeon. The whole life course organization of time for many *chronic* patients, as the descriptive adjective we use for them unwittingly implies, may be organized around dialysis or injections of insulin. Comaroff (1977) has described the battle joined between, among, and inside attenders at clinics and their attendant midwives and doctors over whether about-to-be mothers are well or ill. This too can be seen in terms of time labels: the pregnant for nine months, the expectant mother embedded within a life course, and the in-labour for a period hopefully and usually measured by clock rather than calendar.[7] The analogy but not the congruence with disease, illness, and sickness, respectively, is I think clear, as is the similar linguistic division between the chronic patient, the invalid or cripple, and the disabled.

This draws our attention to a point that Strauss et al. (1985) have made central to their analysis of the modern US hospital. The rarity therein of the acutely sick, combined with the high-technology nature of diagnosis and treatment, means that the knowledge and understanding over time of the sickness trajectory enjoyed by technicians, nurses, and especially patients and their relatives may well be much greater than that of their physicians. In general, the physician may know more than the patient about acute disease in practical as well as in theoretical terms. He or she has seen many discrete patients over a period of years, the chronic patient on the other hand has had the opportunity to study one patient over many years and continuously. A collection of such patients organized into a specific patient group may have much to teach not only about illness and sickness but also about disease, as, at least in the United Kingdom and United States, is now widely professionally recognized.

Albert Kushlick and his colleagues suggested the importance of this long ago (1976) when in evidence to a government committee of enquiry, they suggested that the carers for institutionalized and other incapables could be classified by the time spent with the sufferers. There were, for example, 10 minutes once a week people, two to six hour people, and 12 or 24 hour people. Knowledge should be shared in both directions so that those continuously responsible for life decisions for patients should not only be listened to but also kept fully informed of the latest technical developments in the field. Similarly, 10 minute people needed to learn about the patients' social and personal needs from those in almost continuous contact with them. This was more important than creating, as some had suggested, a new set of professional carers. Since such people were, respectively, relatives, nurses, and physicians, in descending order, Kushlick was assumed to have made a joke in poor taste.

Power, space, and time

Kushlick's suggestion was so serious that it could only, like effective satire, be treated as wit. It draws attention to that creation and control of power through the medium of time which is the core of all cultural performances of sickness. It leads us towards the appreciation of the tragic, because inevitable, contradiction of so-called scientific medicine. Its application depends on the timescale surrounding disease, its efficacy of the timescale surrounding illness. To practise the art of healing, the physician, like the fieldwork-practising anthropologist, meets the sufferer in his or her own time as a coeval. To practise the science of medicine and analyse and treat the disease, the physician distances himself or herself in time from the patient and treats the patient as allochronic, in another time. This is made paradoxically possible by the removal of the patient to hospital, the place that the physician controls but where he or she is not necessarily always co-present in practice although, as we have already seen, is always present in theory. The time transformation is implied in the views on history of Hahn's internist, Barry:

> 'Listen to the patient,' Barry repeats emphatically to the residents. The members of 'the company kept' [i.e., the symptoms] can most often be ascertained from the patient him or herself. 'Nine times out of ten the patient will give you the diagnosis.' [Verbatim quotations from Barry omitted.] Part of what Barry listens to is current symptoms. The remainder is the patient's 'history.' 'Your history is so damned important.... Take that history for what it's worth.' The 'history' is a chronology of the patient's symptoms, activities, and environment. The 'worth' of this chronology, transformed from the patient's to a medical 'history' is essentially diagnostic. This history is cast as an impersonal thing: it is 'that' history and 'your' (the physician's) history, and it is taken by the physician from the patient, medically transformed and medically used.
>
> Again, 'listening to the patient' and 'taking the patient's history' have the appearance of conformity to contemporary concern with the whole person, the patient's interests, individuality, context, and so on. Again the appearance is deceptive. Barry redirects the sharply delimited information drawn from the patient to his physiological examination. 'Listening to the patient' and 'taking the patient's history' are not efforts to sympathetically comprehend the patient's life world, inner meanings, fears or desires, but rather to diagnose disease conceived of by criteria independent of their personal features. (Hahn, 1985: 91)

Our language is more precise than we may give it credit for when we speak of physicians 'taking' rather than 'listening to' patients' histories.[8] This is not the least of the reasons why it is useful to draw attention to the helpfulness of Foucault's analysis of both psychiatry in particular and medicine in general and the relationship of both to the development of society based on both 'discipline' and industry. In particular, he demonstrates that 'The asylum and the hospital are not contingent institutional "contexts" of psychiatry or clinical medicine. They must be included in its definition' (Cousins, 1984).

The cultural performance of sickness involves very specific movements through space and over time, and Foucault (1973) has demonstrated the changed social pattern of this for particular kinds of patient at differing historical periods, just as Goffman (1968) has spelled out the implications of such movements for the individual moral careers of mental hospital and tuberculosis patients, and Turner (1968, 1978) the interactive spiritual perceptions of individuals and collectivities in both African 'cults of affliction' and Marian pilgrimage.

In pre-hospital healing, the sick possess the power of the compelling co-presence of significant others across normal time boundaries. Thus among the Gnau, seriously unwell men move themselves aside from the places where they would be expected to be at particular times and draw attention to their bodies by covering them with dust, and thus by nonverbal departure from norms of space, time, and body surface indicate that they are ill. In many cases that is that, but in others, relatives travel from other villages to be with them at times when they would normally be absent about their own business, or the patient is transported to other places where he would not normally be at that time. Sickness has been thus initiated and its performance, according to circumstances, may or may not be extended into the past by offering explanations of offences against spirits, being in taboo places at taboo times, causing offence to sorcerers, etc.; or into the future by the performance of rites and rituals in addition to the ritual quality of being sick itself, to which Lewis calls attention (1975: 140–1). He sees sickness as a rite of passage, in this case out of society altogether, which he contrasts with Turner's description of some Ndembu sickness performances as making the passage to new status as members of cults of affliction, and with I.M. Lewis's (1971) description of possession by pathogenic spirits as the normal road to a shamanistic calling.

As medical sociologists have partially pointed out, one of the problems of Parsons's concept of the sick role has been its conflation of the direct experience of being ill with the performance of sickness with its associated overlaid performance subroutine of acting as patient. This is one explanation of his readers' perceiving in his work a reduction of Sigerist's social analysis to a psychological one (Frankenberg, 1974).

The power to command the spatial and temporal co-presence of relatives is a common feature of sickness in societies as far apart as the Nyuswa-Zulu (Ngubane, 1977), modern Italy (Frankenberg, 1985), and medieval Jewry, whom the Talmud cautioned against too ready an acceptance of a call to the bedside lest those not sick be encouraged prematurely to enjoy the powers that sickness brings as well as those that it disrupts. It even operates in some hospital systems such as that of Lusaka where in the 1960s it was reported that only cure was offered, care and nurture remaining the responsibility of kin (Boswell, 1965). In those societies that, unlike the Gnau, have full-time healers, these may control the disposition in space and the short periods of co-presence of summoned kin. It is only in industrial society, however, that the continuous sharing of time, day and night, by patients and their relatives is overridden for long or short periods by medical staff.

Even there, as we have seen, it is restored by impending death or birth, or by belief in the rights and duties of the nuclear family in conjunction with the need for continuous care beyond the time resources of staff (as in modern UK paediatric and labour wards).

The control over where the patient is at what time and over who is co-present with her or him is well described in A.E. Ellis's fictionalized account of his experiences immediately after the Second World War in an alpine tuberculosis sanatorium in Haute Savoie (1958).

The major mechanism of this control, so vital to the maintenance of the power relations that first bring patients to the hospital and then make sure that they conform, is the control of patients' time. One of the most perceptive subjective accounts of this is, unsurprisingly, that of Oliver Sacks (1984), who, as he reminds us, was a doctor for 15 years before becoming a patient, and a patient who from the point of view of hospital staff was unnecessarily and impertinently concerned with his own time and his control over it. After his account of the de-personalizing admission procedures, 'One is no longer a person – one is now an inmate. One understands that this is protective, but it is quite dreadful too' (Sacks, 1984: 28), he records his delighted surprise at being addressed by his name by a nurse and thus rehumanized, and then the less pleasant first experience of having a 'history' taken from him rather than by him. This produced the worries common to patients and self-reflexive students of E.H. Carr and Braudel about what might be relevant let alone salient. The relatively junior doctors who question Sacks tell him he is to have a general anaesthetic for the necessary exploration next day and when he protested:

> They said, no, general anesthesia was the rule in such cases, and besides (they smiled) the surgeons wouldn't want me talking or asking questions all through the operation!
> I wanted to pursue the point, but there was something in their tone and manner that made be desist. (ibid: 29)

He decided to exercise what he still saw as peer rights and talk to Swan, his surgeon, the following morning. After arranging his affairs by phone and after a good night's sleep, he awoke at 5.00, and remembered that the operation was scheduled for 9.30, and his unaccustomed viewpoint on the time drama was resumed:

> I waited eagerly for Swan to come. Six o'clock, seven o'clock, eight o'clock.... Wasn't he coming, I asked Sister, a formidable-looking woman in severe dark blue (the jolly staff-nurse of the night before had been in a striped uniform).
> 'Mr. Swan will come when he pleases,' she said tartly. (ibid: 30)

At 8.30 he gets his preoperative injections from a nurse and at 8.45 he rings to ask what he had been given. He reports that after the injection he had not taken his eyes off his watch: 'Mr. Swan made his appearance at 8.53 and found me gazing at my watch' (ibid.: 30).

The surgeon turned out to be hearty rather than helpful and the familiar 'How are we doing today?' and 'Nothing to worry about!' were more or less communicated on the run with other clichés. Sacks rang the bell again for the now obviously impatient sister:

> 'What is it?' she said. 'Why have you called me?'
>
> 'Mr. Swan,' I said, enunciating my words carefully. 'He didn't stay very long. He was just in and out. He seemed to be in an awful hurry.'
>
> 'Well, I never,' Sister huffed. 'He's a very busy man. You're lucky he looked in at all.' (ibid.: 31)

Dr Sacks continued to be concerned with the slipping away of his control over time through the characteristic counting away of consciousness imposed by the anaesthetist; his final conscious memory of complaining, apparently correctly, that the second hand of the preparation room clock had stuck; to awakening to tell a houseman that a few minutes ago his knee had felt fine and discovering that seven hours had passed; and lastly to 48 hours of semiconsciousness. At one stage he does recall his experiences as a new boy at school and compare himself to a prisoner. His knowledge and former status enable him, notwithstanding the linguistic shift from Swan to Mr Swan, in some sense to distance himself and thus to prolong resistance beyond that possible to those totally encompassed within the system.

Julius Roth, distanced by being 'A Yank in the NHS' (1977)[9] is also able to give us an insight into the way that control over the situation of the patient in space and time creates and reinforces general patterns of control.

No disease was in fact involved, nor did anyone feel ill. The case was merely that Roth, his wife, and son were all agreed that the son, Timothy, should not participate in outdoor games at school. An aspect of British culture unfamiliar to them was that such a decision was only possible if medically legitimated. Even in the absence of disease and illness, the cultural performance of sickness in some societies and at some times is required. The performance began by making an appointment at the group practice of which they were registered patients, where they were by chance seen by a trainee general practitioner (GP) who took a comprehensive history and referred them to a consultant. Two weeks later they responded to a postal summons to attend the outpatient department of the local hospital, where the consultant took an even more elaborate history, performed a detailed physical examination, and arranged for urine and blood tests and a chest X-ray, which he insisted had to be done as an inpatient for, it was thought by the patient and his father, two days. Another letter and several weeks later, Timothy was admitted on a Sunday evening to the Royal Infirmary, although, of course, no tests were scheduled until the following day. Roth rather tartly comments on the later frank explanation of the consultant that this was for the bureaucratic convenience of the hospital staff. He was kept in hospital for five days, to the detriment, Roth maintains, of the accuracy of at least some of the tests. Nothing was found to be the matter and it was concluded, as the parents and son had always maintained, that the reasons for not participating were 'psychological', although the latter declined to take up the offer of psychiatric treatment or to enforce consumption of the tranquilizers provided, and persisted in their request for a note to the school. The consultant said that it was not possible for him to provide such a note but that he would write with a recommendation to that effect to the GP. So several weeks after the first request, they were once more in the GP's office and a letter was written and the boy excused from all games (not merely outdoor games as had originally be requested), with only relatively minor harassment and comparatively few further school-imposed visits to the doctor to confirm the continuance of the legitimated excuse.

Roth (1977: 193) analyses this experience in terms of the inappropriate power attributed to the medical profession by the refusal of other agencies, in this case the school and its staff, to take responsibility for their own decisions; the redefinition of clients' requests and the use of power to make their definition definitive; the control of information; the provision of rigidly defined facilities that have to be accepted by clients; and the use of centralization to cut clients off from alternatives. Rather surprisingly, given that he originated the topic of time in medical settings (Roth, 1963; Roth and Douglas, 1983), he does not draw attention to the temporal aspects of his account.

The sensitized reader is, however, aware of the following:

1 The deterrent delay induced by the school authorities' reference to the health services, which might well have discouraged a less resolute family.
2 The fact that transactions with the GP were by appointment at his place and time and, as it happened, with someone early in his career (and thus perhaps himself more likely to evade responsibility by referring on).
3 The central role of the history at the expense of the present situation and future possibilities (an aspect to which I return in a later section, p. 18–21).
4 The control of the patient's person through transfer to a place where his time was no longer his own. (See the discussion of history-taking above, p. 11).

Such subjection was clearly not biomedically necessary in this case, but Roth argues, somewhat contradictorily to the medically qualified Sacks, that it is usually not and perhaps is never necessary in other cases either. Since it was for most purposes common ground that no disease was present and there was certainly no threat to life either, the normal trade-off of tolerating a long wait for a short interview since life itself might be thereby prolonged did not here apply.

Hahn's Barry Siegler had to turn would-be patients away despite the fact that they were paying, had the choice of other doctors, and had sometimes, by his own account, to wait two to three hours in his office for their average 12.3 minutes. Presumably they knew that he worked through the day without lunch to fit them in, and hoped, sometimes correctly, that his obsession with anticoagulants and his general treatments would prolong their lives (Hahn, 1985: 70 and passim). The case study of Siegler reveals very vividly a time organization of medicine that would be absurdly irrational if all that was at issue was a kind of patient care analogous either to other forms of concern for the individual or even to the care of mechanisms that have gone wrong. We are not surprised to learn that physicians' time is organized differently from that of either priests or motor mechanics. That does not necessarily make it ideal for healing people.

Roth's failure to utilize the insights about time that he has taught to the rest of us also has profound political implications. It is perhaps the reason why his remedies learned from some aspects of the women's movement, like Anselm Strauss's, are merely radical rather than revolutionary in that they offer hope but combine it with despair. Despairing of fundamental reform of the physician or formal service organizations, their hope comes through self-help organizations, consumer education, and patients being accompanied by advocates. Revolutionary changes in health services, like those elsewhere, require that time itself is turned upside down. The message of Marx's *Capital* to workers, that they should take charge of their own time, whether it is interpreted in terms of state socialism or cooperation, applies also to patients.

Adults in industrial society, outside the hospital, do, albeit within a framework of publicly scheduled events (such as opening hours, times of performance, transport timetables, programme times, etc.), organize their own time in their own places, but they have it organized for them in places where they are constrained by work or public regulation. Such places of constraint include, of course, the home as the locus of child care and care for the elderly and infirm. Classical (Jahoda, et al., 1972) and recent studies of male unemployment suggest that uncertainty of time scheduling is, after an initial period of the enjoyment of time anarchy, the first major problem to be resolved. Removal of patients, whether male or female, to hospital or even to clinics, whether outpatient departments of hospital or consulting rooms of GPs, puts them in a space where the patients' uncertainty is reinforced by the certitudes of the physician's (and to a lesser extent other health workers') understanding of complicated routines. Paradoxically, when the timing of events such as release from a long-stay mental hospital, or in the past, tuberculosis sanatorium, is almost as uncertain for the staff as it is for the patient, this too becomes a means of social control through real or apparent powers to make it less so. This is a major theme in literature, in both Ellis's *The Rack* (1958) and Mann's *The Magic Mountain* (1960), as well as in sociology, in Julian Roth's *Timetables* (1963) and as part of more complex analyses in Goffman's *Asylums* (1968) and Davis's and Horobin's conclusion to *Medical Encounters* (1977). In all these works we read of patients' attempts to reduce the uncertain timing of future events by wresting from physicians the knowledge of probabilities or by inventing certainty and progress by devising ways of literally 'marking' time (Davis and Horobin, 1977: 217–18). It is one of the reasons that militant nurses in the United States are claiming the right, at present held exclusively by physicians, to fix the date of patient's discharge.

We can then develop Kushlick's classification by contact time with patients in another way, by looking at tense in the discourse of healing. As we saw in Sacks's anxieties about the salience of events in his personal history, entry into clinical control does not merely imply power over the sufferer's present but also over his or her past and, as we have just seen, future. In Kushlick's terms, the agent who is least present, the physician, has the power to re-present the past and the future. The nursing staff, whose presents are long but fragmented, normally control only segments of the now. The 24 hour people, whether patients themselves or their relatives, while their omnipresents theoretically give them power over time – past, present and future – are in practice rendered anachronous by uncertainty. Being made to wait and not knowing what is to happen and when is not an incidental of the cultural performance of sickness in biomedicine-dominated healing, it is central to the conversion of the suffering to the patient, what Zola (1973) called the pathway from the person to the patient. In the terms of Fabian (1983), to whose characterization of anthropology I am about to turn, it is the way that medicine creates its other and makes its object. Conversely, a medicine that saw other health workers, let alone the patients, as equal participants in the healing process would neither need nor be able to treat the time of others as within its control. If Strauss et al. (1985) are correct in their diagnosis of the nature of both disease and its effective treatment in modern urban industrial society, namely, that the former is chronic and the latter is high-tech, there is in

fact no other rational choice. To achieve their goals, hospital physicians, at least, have to share decision-making not only with other
health workers and technicians (present in the hospital or not) but also
with patients and their significant others. The very recognition of this
necessity would transform biomedical treatment into a more complex
form of social healing, as already happens in some hospices and
paediatric units. I, however, share the more pessimistic/optimistic
view of Marx that those who hold power do not necessarily relinquish
it merely because they can no longer exercise it effectively. Historical
changes, like women in labour, still need midwives, even if for both
they can most usefully be chosen from among their friends.

The tragic contradiction: in our time and in theirs

Johannes Fabian in a stimulating and important book (1983), which
forces us to regard anthropology in an entirely new light, draws
attention to the significant peculiarity of the ethnographic present.
Social and cultural anthropologists, unlike most other social scientists
and all historians, usually or often live alongside and share the
experiences of those they study and whose society or aspects of whose
society they intend to analyse. They become coeval with them while
they collect their material. The anthropological exercise, however, also
involves the scholar in relieving the experience in his or her mind and
re-presenting it in speech and in print for an audience other than those
who were the subjects. Paradoxically, if we follow Fabian's argument,
the anthropologist by present-ing his or her material in the present
tense freezes the past in a way that establishes the other-timeworld-
liness, the allochronicity, of those who were studied. The present tense,
Fabian argues, is a signal identifying a discourse in an observer's
language. It separates observer from observed; the observer has moved
on, usually to another place as well as to another time. The observed
remain crystallized in space and time.

I tell my students that the Dinka *are* raided by the Nuer and
absorbed into their lineages; unless the students are unusually alert,
they do not realize that I am talking about what Evans-Pritchard
thought that he could deduce from his observations in 1930 and 1935–6
and finally published in 1940 when I was 10 years old and my students'
parents were perhaps as yet unborn. Neither my students nor I would
normally, as anthropologists, make a connection between those political events in the British Empire (the bombing of Nuer herds and
settlements) to which Evans-Pritchard does refer in the past tense and
the realities of the Nuer past and their famine- and civil war-haunted
present (August 1986). Interestingly enough, it is precisely when
looking at Evans-Pritchard's classic analysis of Nuer time reckoning

(1939), that one becomes most conscious of the effect of this way of thinking about the other. For here, and in the chapter on the same topic that substantially repeats it in *The Nuer* (1940), Evans-Pritchard makes the classical anthropological error of comparing the informal behaviour of the other with the formal of the self. The Nuer, when Evans-Pritchard studied them, saw time in structural and 'oecological' terms and had no clocks.[10] In Oxford, the clock and the history-book chronology were present but perhaps not omnipresent. In their spare time, even Fellows of All Souls may also have found it less difficult to discuss time with the Nuer than Evans-Pritchard supposed. Gellner pointed out long ago: 'how very general considerations, which in the past have arisen from analysing the relation between thought and things as such, have entered anthropological theory in the misleading guise of something specifically intimately connected with anthropological material' (1958: 183).

It is no wonder that anthropologists bringing their discipline back home to Western Europe and the United States feel sufficiently uncomfortable to write and confer frequently about the epistemological problems and to seek to study what exotic other they can find even in their own countries[11] or to study the near at hand and to present it as other. Such discussions have led to the advocacy of a more self-reflexive approach to the interpretation of fieldwork experience, which as Fabian argues implies the representation to ourselves and others of our own past. Furthermore, if this intersubjectivity is to extend beyond fellow anthropologists, we must, he suggests, be able to share each other's past in order to be knowingly in each other's presence.

Anthropologists can perhaps all too readily empathize with physicians. For some at least of these latter are faced with the problem that in order to get to know their patients they must be co-present with them as people in so fundamental a way as to be described as coevals. Paul Atkinson (1981) has amusingly and in another sense tragically described how, on a shorter timescale, clinical teachers present the past symptoms of their successfully treated patients in the present tense. When patients have the temerity somatically or verbally to deny what is being demonstrated, they are reminded that physical and social coevalness are not identical. However, it is always important to distinguish between physicians involved in primary care and physicians operating as specialists. An analogy may be drawn with the division in the United Kingdom's other senior profession between solicitor and barrister. The former, like the GP, knows the circumstances of the client/patient in all their temporal and spatial density. The latter, like the specialist, puts the client's case in the context of the allochronic law court.

A primary health care physician, the GP in Britain, ideally and sometimes in practice, does not so much take a history (past) as take a present of the patient's social, psychological being.[12] It has been suggested that, in practice, GPs prescribe at this moment when the physician is nearest to achieving present (coeval) empathy with the patient (Howie, 1984). In scientific theory, however, what physicians should do at this point is to diagnose, that is to say, to withdraw their attention from the patients' social being (and by implication becoming) and turn it towards the patient's body and the biological processes to which it is, more or less passively, subject. Hahn's Barry Siegler, half GP, half consultant physician, is very conscious of the contradiction and speaks of his patient's problem as a 'picture', a 'story', a 'thing' (Hahn, 1985: 79). Living past/present becomes biomedical notional present tense: 'You have been overdoing it... exposed to infection etc. etc.... You have caught, developed X... but... X is, it has these characteristics.'

Although Sassall does certainly get closer to his patients (or perhaps Berger is a romantic to Hahn's realist), in the end even he comes back to biology, the body, and a named disease:

> The doctor in order to recognize the illness fully – I say fully because the recognition must be such as to indicate the specific treatment – must first recognize the patient as a person: but for the patient – provided that he trusts the doctor and that trust finally depends on the efficacy of his treatment – the doctor's recognition of his illness is a help because it separates and depersonalizes that illness. (Berger, 1967: 68)

and again:

> No, he is acknowledged as a good doctor because he meets the deep but unformulated expectation of the sick for a sense of fraternity. He recognizes them. Sometimes he fails – often because he has missed a critical opportunity and the patient's suppressed resentment becomes too hard to break through – but there is about him the constant will of a man trying to recognize. (ibid.: 70–1)

and finally:

> When patients are describing their conditions or worries to Sassall, instead of nodding his head or murmuring 'yes,' he says again and again 'I know,' 'I know.' He says it with genuine sympathy. Yet it is what he says whilst he is wanting to know more. He already knows what it is like to be this patient in a certain condition: but he does not yet know the full explanation of that condition, nor the extent of his own power. (ibid.: 74)

If general medicine is concerned with the present tense, specialties present surprising and paradoxical tenses. Thus surgery speaks to the future: 'You will be better when I have removed the growth, the limb'. The most dramatic example is cosmetic plastic surgery that changes the present by creating a future from which part of the evidence of the past has disappeared. Psychiatry, however, at least in so far as it is based on psychotherapy, makes the extension of the present into the future bearable by permitting the restructuring of the past. In fact Bloch suggests that the great betrayal of Freud and Jung arose from their neglect of daydreams, aspirations to a better future, in order to concentrate on night dreams, a distorted presentation of an unhappy past. He marginally prefers Freud who, although he wrongly saw daydreams as mere stepping stones to those of the night (1986: 86), at least tries to overcome the effects of the past on the material lives of his patients, whereas Jung, according to Bloch, merely tries to situate his patients' immaterial psyches permanently not only in their own pasts but also in the mythical past of all humankind (1986, vol. I: 51–113).

Bloch is angered by this because he sees in it the denial of what is to him the most important of human emotions, namely hope, which he sees as pointing to the future, and since he is a materialist, to the future of the socially situated body. It is with this last that the medical usage of time – past, present, and future – is ultimately concerned.

Crossing frontiers: time and the hospitalized body

It is of course an absurd truism to state that when patients are moved to hospital they are accompanied by their bodies, but there is nevertheless a necessity when discussing medicine and time to emphasize this. In fact, in Goffman's celebrated discussion of the admission procedures to long-stay institutions (1968), which are in many ways similar to hospital procedure, he emphasizes the stripping off of integuments including clothing and supposed surface dirt, in order that the outsider, stripped of clothes and roles, may be reclothed as the first stage to socialization as an inmate. Second, Foucault has drawn attention to the discipline of the body exemplified in the rule of St Benedict and other monastic codes, the introduction and development of military drill, and methods of mass production in industry. Both Goffman and Foucault draw attention not only to the spatial but also the temporal implications of these trends; thus inmates of total institutions like those modelled by Goffman are always constrained to rise, retire, and eat at fixed times, and monasteries, barracks, and mass-production factories impose a rigid timetable on the body movements of those permanently or temporarily confined within them. Building on, developing, and sometimes criticizing these ideas, Armstrong (1983), Giddens (1984), and Bryan S. Turner (1984) have severally been able theoretically to illuminate the relationships between power, social organization, and the use and perception of the body, as in an earlier period did Mary Douglas (1973) inspired by Mauss (1936).

What I want to argue here is that relatively short-term and thera-

peutic rather than custodial hospitalization is concerned with the body
neither in its 'normal' socially constructed form nor as a totally
biological entity. It is nearer to the latter and, as I have argued,
biomedical models of sickness performance demand that this should
be so. Nevertheless, especially at moments of loss of, or return to,
consciousness or of material flow across or through body boundaries,
the breach of cultural norm obstructs the acceptance of the body's
'purely' biological nature even within the bounds of hospital anti-
temporality. If we accept Mary Douglas's view that the natural body
and the social body reproduce and reinforce the reciprocal images of
one another, then the removal of the patient's body to the hospital
implies more than its biological reshaping. In fact, the total cultural
performance of biomedical healing is concerned neither with social
persons nor with natural physiological or pathological processes but
precisely with transitions between the two. The hospital body and the
embodied patient are seen as bounded, and what has to be controlled
are movements within and across those boundaries. In this control,
time is the essential factor.

In private life patients may or may not have been 'regular' in their
habits; hospital routine tries to ensure that they are. Cartwright (1964:
69) optimistically interprets this: 'the strangeness of a new environment is succeeded by the security of a known routine'. We have seen
something of Roth's view, argued also by many others, that notwithstanding the power of the organization and its certain (because
fixed) temporal and other routines, the outcome of hospital order is a
negotiated one, but one in which the patient negotiates from a position
of temporal disruption and uncertainty. Ailon Shiloh's study of
hospital patients in Israel led her to conclude that a bipolar distribution
of patients existed in the hospital that she studied: those who saw
themselves as partners to the staff (equalitarian) and those who saw
themselves as acted upon (hierarchical) (1972). Both groups of patients
were: 'prompt to reply, were articulate and replete with details as to the
nature and cause of their pre-hospitalized condition at the very time
that they were hesitant, brief and vague as to the treatment and
prognosis aspects of their condition within the hospital.'

I am not, of course, suggesting that this is deliberately organized to
give power to staff. It is merely a side-effect of the focus upon, and the
social and temporal restructuring of, transitions across the boundaries
of the body.

The day's first such transition, which differs from the others in that
material does not pass, is that from sleep to consciousness. In British
hospitals, at least, the day starts early, and although Cartwright's
study appeared over 20 years ago (1964), a hospital recently portrayed
on television in which patients were asked when they would like to be

woken was presented as an exception. In Cartwright's sample, 95 per cent of the patients were woken before 7.00 a.m., 62 per cent before 6.00 a.m. and 35 per cent before 5.30 a.m. Although many patients saw the nurses' point of view and none mentioned being awoken early directly as a reason for feeling critical of nurses, patients who were awakened early were in fact those most critical of nurses (Cartwright, 1964: 38–9).

The Royal Commission report of 1979 (Merrison, 1979) also drew critical attention to unnecessary early waking, attributing it to tradition, the 'Nightingale' ward design, and putting the convenience of the staff before that of the patients.[13] The Royal Commission explains the 'necessity' by the timing of shift changeover, itself dependent on the availability of public transport; medical rounds; medicine rounds; and the need to collect laboratory specimens. (They might have mentioned also the necessity of providing the patients with regular meals at relatively fixed times with limited staff.) All except the first of these (shift changes) involve a departure from 'normal' patterns of crossings of body apertures and translating of body fluids from outside to inside as well as extrabody substances in the other direction. Fluids leave at the wrong time, the wrong place, and in the presence of the wrong significant others. In the Nightingale wards, the specifics of shame are hidden by the screens around the bed; the generalities, by the hospital's time out of life. The rigid time structures of the hospital emphasize the anti-temporality of the experience in relation to 'normal' worldly time, in just the same way as the formality and timed ritual of the pilgrimage at Lough Dergh, for example (Turner and Turner, 1978: chapter III). Thomas Mann's *The Magic Mountain* (1960) presents a set of variations on this theme for the extreme case of the long-stay tuberculosis sanatorium. Senior physicians, however, are less protected since, as we have already seen, they are at once privileged and condemned to breach both sacred and profane time boundaries, as well as licensed and required to penetrate those of the body. Such a view helps us to understand the contradictions in Barry Siegler's combination of compassion and sexist vulgarity expressed in his own words and reported by Hahn (1985: 103–6).

Hahn argues that two idiomatic strands pervade the way Barry talks about his work: an image of the body and of the dynamics of flow and obstruction with it. His movements about the hospital, Hahn sees in a similar way: 'Barry is perpetually concerned with the qualities of channels of passage, with obstructions to passage, and with rates and regularities of flow' (ibid.: 104). These are charted for the patient who is visualized as a ship at sea. His favourite medicament, as we have already noted, is the anticoagulant and he is also vitally concerned with his own unobstructed flow through hospital corridors and overcrowded streets to keep the appointments on his overcrowded schedule. A similar imagery is applied to his efforts and those of others to keep patients flowing to and from treatment departments of the hospital and in and out of the hospital itself. It is, however, when things go wrong or are obstructed that Barry turns to scatological and aggressive, sadistic, sexual metaphor, unthinkable for Berger's Sassall or in extra-hospital practice generally. Patients and others are seen as turds or shits and Barry 'may tangle ass holes with them'. Things he disagrees with or is ambivalent about 'need to be screwed' and he makes full use of the love/hate ambiguity of cant terms for the sexual act. As Hahn gently comments: 'Engagement with his patients' bodies touches him in a personal, emotional way. Beyond his medical concern for proper flow within the body, Barry is troubled by body effluence and excretion. Here the concern is one of contamination – contamination not in a medical sense, but in a more generic sense of dirt and impurity' (ibid.: 105–6).

Hahn has earlier described Barry's moral disapproval and contempt – 'If you give a woman a vaginal suppository, you've got to tell her to take the foil off' (ibid.: 103) – of those he thinks of as promiscuous, the alcoholic, and those who make their diabetes, for example, worse by their eating habits. In other words, those who do not suitably control their body boundaries. Unsurprisingly, given what Hahn has told us about Barry's religious background and beliefs, this disapproval is extended especially to women who, in the Christian as well as the Jewish tradition in which Barry has been socialized, are a particular threat to the clear maintenance of the timing of cultural natural boundaries. Both Jewish and Catholic concern with sexual intercourse and time of the menstrual month testifies to this concern. His attitudes to young women (whether patients or nurses; there is no direct evidence of his attitude to young women doctors) is in sharp contrast to his attitude to his favourite patients, no longer sexually or boundary-threatening 'little old ladies'. Apart from any personal idiosyncrasy of Hahn's subject, I would wish to suggest that the scheduling and lack of boundaries of Barry's time means that he is not protected as are other members of the hospital staff from the continual culturally uncontrolled natural breaches of body boundaries to which they are all subjected. At the same time he, alongside other physicians, has the power, the time, the captive subordinate audience, and the licensed places in which to spell out his sadistic fantasies. Not all physicians indulge their opportunities as does Barry, but in the United Kingdom and the United States most have the same structural milieu. The nature of the jokes in the US-produced 'MASH' and the popular UK medical television comedies and films suggest a rich vein for cultural anthropological mining.

Conclusion

In this chapter I have merely begun to explore the interrelations of biological and social time in the cultural performance of sickness, especially when healing is based on a biomedical mode. In some ways this is in fact the most interesting model to study since biomedical physicians and other health workers share an ideology of curing a disease: that is, restoring or reconstituting a biological status quo. The stark choice of death or restoration to health leaves them little room for utopian visions (Bloch, 1986, vol. II: 467) or social fantasies such as might be indulged by benevolent African traditional healers cleansing a village of sickness-causing witchcraft or sorcery, or even malevolent Californian politicians seeking to rid the world of sin, homosexuality, AIDS, and their own unacknowledged, repressed temptations all at one stroke. I have found in the scholarly literature only hints of the different time worlds of old and young, male and female, rich and poor, dying and recovering patients, and their similarly stratified doctors, nurses, and therapists. I have had to have recourse, without great reluctance, to the fictionalized or 'unscientific' accounts of sick doctors and recovered sociologists and novelists.

Nevertheless it seems to me clear that this particular approach is revealing. In the mainstream of societies such as the United Kingdom and United States, the cultural performance of sickness within a biomedical framework takes place in a context where social, and especially temporal, mechanisms to control relationships of nature and culture are disrupted. In order to maintain social order and restore natural order, patients are removed from their normal temporalities to a space where the time view of others can be imposed upon them. This is not incidental to, but an integral part of, the *modus operandi* of biomedicine as at present practised, hence my suggestion of tragic inevitability. It iatrogenetically produces a situation of enhanced power for the healers and reduced autonomy for the patients, notwithstanding the latter's attempts to negotiate their own reconstituted temporalities. As Oakley (1979, 1980) and other writers, as well as the recent experience of Wendy Savage (1986) in Britain have shown, and as we may well have experienced as parents, unsurprisingly if my analysis is correct, the contradiction of temporalities and of aspects of body boundaries is sharpest between social and natural motherhood on the one side and class- and gender-constructed obstetric medicine on the other. The designation of pregnancy as pregnancy rather than expectant motherhood, and also as disease, is a move in a power struggle in which the conceptualizing of women's and of health workers' time is of central importance. As every English schoolchild used to know, the fact that authority may sincerely believe itself to be acting in the interest of the subject does not detract from its exercise of power or from the stimulus to opposition.

But in Western medicine in general, time is more important as the basis of power and control than merely as the basis of value (important though Ricardo and Marx showed that to be in general). The problems that this creates for both patients and healers are not necessarily different in the totally capitalistic medicine of the United States, the partially socialized medicine of the United Kingdom, or the totally socialized medicine of the Soviet Union. The more that China turns to bureaucratized, urban, curative, hospital biomedicine, the sharper will problems there become. Where diverse systems do differ is both in their capacity to resolve such issues without the total rejection of biomedical practice, and in the relevance for them of its creating, maintaining, and reinforcing the central ideological tenets of the society. These last are the two major overriding problems that require solution through social practice rather than mere research or scholarly presentation.

Notes

The article contained in this chapter first appeared in the *International Journal of Health Services*, 18(1), 1988. I am grateful to Michael Young and participants in the 1986 Association for the Social Study of Time conference at Dartington for encouragement and constructive criticism of a preliminary presentation. I am especially grateful to Pauline Hunt and Ruth Frankenberg who read the whole of an earlier draft and made many helpful suggestions. My other debts are all too evident in the text.

1. The general point is made by Goffman, 1968.

2. 'coupling constraints' (Giddens, 1984: 114).

3. I use the term illth as I did in an earlier paper (Frankenberg, 1986: 603) in preference to ill-being used in earlier times by Herbert Spencer and Carlyle. Illth was used in the late nineteenth century by Ruskin, Sir Oliver Lodge, and George Bernard Shaw as an antonym to wealth in the sense of well-being and as a subheading in the original Fabian Essays. I use it to mean the converse of health, an expression of dis-ease.

4. 'Emic' and 'etic' are terms of art introduced into anthropology by Marvin Harris and now widely current in the discipline to that of the subjects of study. The latter to an interpretation inserted into the theoretical framework of the observer/analyst and his or her colleagues.

5. For a further critical discussion of this and other categorizations see Hahn (1980).

6. I have introduced these concepts in an earlier paper (Frankenberg, 1987) seeking to operationalize Heidegger's concept of 'life-towards-death' (Baumann, 1978). Most empirical sociologists who have taken an interest at all in such topics have concentrated on deathhandying conceived as one word. On the one hand, this feeds the illusion that all but the final stages of the life course can reasonably be analysed without reference to its universal and inevitable end; on the other, it leaves the problem to hospice workers and specialist social scientists. Lifedeath is used in place of that part of life in which death is part of what Bloch (1986) calls the not yet conscious. Deathlife is used to indicate that part of life which is lived in the consciousness of its not too far distant end.

7. See Rosengren and DeVault (1963) for an analysis of the use of space, barriers and lighting to mark the boundaries of microperiods within the longer time periods of medicalized labour in a hospital setting.

8. Pauline Hunt has pointed out to me the similarity between this and industrial situations in which workers' views on policy are sought, apparently listened to, and then either not acted upon or used in an alien management context.

9. See also especially Rosemary Firth's and Ann Holohan's papers in the same volume (Firth, 1977; Holohan, 1977).

10. In Masai tourist villages in Kenya in the 1980s, the proprietors made sure that the 'primitives' on display hid their wrist watches and transistor radios during visiting times (Bruner and Kirshenblatt-Gimblett, 1985).

11. See Jackson (1986), and especially Ardener's (1986) article therein.

12. It is instructive to compare the view and practice of Hahn's anthropologically intuited Barry Siegler with Berger's (1967) poetically evoked Sassal, the English country doctor of *A Fortunate Man*.

13. It did not draw attention to Cartwright's finding that the situation of teaching hospitals was better, probably because not only were there more nurses but they also worked a three-shift instead of a two-shift system (Cartwright, 1964: 171).

References

Ardener, E. (1986) 'Remote areas: Some theoretical considerations', in A. Jackson (ed.), *Anthropology at Home*. Associations of Social Anthropologists Monograph 25. London: Tavistock Press. pp. 38–54.

Armstrong, D. (1983) *Political Anatomy of the Body: Medical Knowledge in Britain in the Twentieth Century*. Cambridge: Cambridge University Press.

Armstrong, D. (1984) 'The patient's view', *Social Science and Medicine*, 18(9): 737–44.

Armstrong, D. (1985) 'Space and time in British general practice', *Social Science and Medicine*, 20(7): 659–66.

Atkinson, P. (1981) 'Time and cool patients', in P. Atkinson and C. Heath (eds), *Medical Work: Realities and Routines*. Farnborough: Gower. pp. 41–54.

Baumann, Z. (1978) *Hermeneutics and Social Science: Approaches to Understanding*. London: Hutchinson University Library. p. 165.

Berger, J. (1967) *A Fortunate Man: The Story of a Country Doctor*. London: Allen Lane, The Penguin Press.

Bloch, E. (1986) *The Principle of Hope*, vols I, II, III. Oxford: Blackwell.

Bloor, D.C. (1976) *Knowledge and Social Imagery*. London: Routledge and Kegan Paul.

Bluebond-Langner, M. (1978) *The Private Worlds of Dying Children*. Princeton, N.J.: Princeton University Press.

Boswell, D.M. (1965) *Escorts of Hospital Patients: A Preliminary Report on a Social Survey Undertaken at Lusaka Central Hospital from July to August 1964*. Rhodes Livingstone Communication 29. Lusaka, Zambia.

Bruner, E. and Kirshenblatt-Gimblett, B. (1985) 'Tourist performance and the ethnographic original'. Presented at the American Anthropology Association annual conference, Washington DC.

Cartwright, A. (1964) *Human Relations and Hospital Care*. London: Routledge and Kegan Paul.

Collier, P. and Horowitz, D. (1985) *The Kennedys: An American Drama*, London: Pan Books. p. 540.

Comaroff, J. (1977) 'Conflicting paradigms of pregnancy: Managing ambiguity in antenatal encounters', in A. Davis and G. Horobin (eds), *Medical Encounters: The Experience of Illness and Treatment*. London: Croom Helm. pp. 115–34.

Comaroff, J. (1982) 'Medicine: Symbol and ideology', in P. Wright and A. Treacher (eds), *The Problem of Medical Knowledge: Examining the Social Construction of Medicine*. Edinburgh: Edinburgh University Press. pp. 49–68.

Cousins, M. and Hussain, A. (1984) *Michel Foucault*. London: Macmillan. p. 76.

Davis, A. and Horobin, G. (eds) (1977) *Medical Encounters: The Experience of Illness and Treatment*. London: Croom Helm.

Douglas, M. (1973) *Natural Symbols*. Harmondsworth: Penguin Books.

Ellis, A.E. (1958) *The Rack*. Harmondsworth: Penguin Books.

Evans-Pritchard, E.E. (1939) 'Nuer time reckoning', *Africa*, 12(2): 189–216.

Evans-Pritchard, E.E. (1940) *The Nuer*. Oxford: Clarendon Press.

Fabian, J. (1983) *Time and the Other*. New York: Columbia University Press.

Firth, R. (1977) 'Routines in a tropical diseases hospital', in A. Davis and G. Horobin (eds), *Medical Encounters: The Experience of Illness and Treatment*. London: Croom Helm. pp. 143–58.

Foucault, M. (1973) *The Birth of the Clinic: An Archaeology of Medical Perception*. New York: Pantheon Press.

Frankenberg, R. (1974) 'Functionalism and after? Theory and developments in social science applied to the health field', *International Journal of Health Services*, 4(3): 411–27.

Frankenberg, R. (1985) 'Malattia Come Festa: Sickness as Celebration and Socialisation: Children's Accounts of Sickness Episodes in a Tuscan Community', Conference paper, Keele.

Frankenberg, R. (1986) 'Sickness as cultural performance: Drama, trajectory and pilgrimage. Root metaphors and the making of social disease', *International Journal of Health Services*, 16(4): 603–26.

Frankenberg, R. (1987) 'Life: Cycle, trajectory, or pilgrimage? A social production approach to Marxism, metaphor and mortality', in A. Bryman et al. (eds), *Rethinking the Life Cycle*. London: Macmillan.

Frankenberg, R. and Leeson, J. (1976) 'Disease, illness and sickness: Aspects of the choice of healer in a Lusaka suburb', in J. Loudon (ed.), *Social Anthropology and Medicine*, Association of Social Anthropologists Monograph 13. London and New York: Academic Press.

Gabbay, J. (1982) 'Asthma attacked? Tactics for the reconstruction of a disease concept', in P. Wright and A. Treacher (eds), *The Problem of Medical Knowledge: Examining the Social Construction of Medicine*. Edinburgh: Edinburgh University Press. pp. 23–48.

Gellner, E. (1958) 'Time and theory in social anthropology', *Mind*, 67: 182–202.

Giddens, A. (1984) *The Constitution of Society*. Cambridge: Polity Press.

Goffman, E. (1968) *Asylums: Essays on the Social Situation of Mental Patients and other Inmates*. Harmondsworth: Penguin Books.

Hahn, R.A. (1980) 'Rethinking "illness" and "disease" ', *Contributions to Asian Studies*, XVIII: 1–23.

Hahn, R.A. (1985) 'A world of internal medicine: Portrait of an internist', in R.A. Hahn and A.D. Gaines (eds), *Physicians of Western Medicine: Anthropological Approaches to Theory and Practice*. Dordrecht: Reidel, pp. 51–111.

Holohan, A. (1977) 'Diagnosis: The end of transition', in A. Davis and G. Horobin (eds), *Medical Encounters: The Experience of Illness and Treatment*. London: Croom Helm. pp. 87–97.

Howie, J.G.R. (1984) 'Research in general practice: Pursuit of knowledge or defence of wisdom', *British Medical Journal*, 289: 1770–2.

Jackson, A. (1986) *Anthropology at Home*. Association of Social Anthropologists Monograph 25. London: Tavistock Press.

Jahoda, M., Lazarsfeld, P.F. and Zeisel, H. (1972) *Marienthal*. London: Tavistock Press. (First published 1933.)

Kleinman, A. (1978) 'Concepts and a model for the comparison of medical systems as cultural systems', *Social Science and Medicine*, 12(2B): 85–93.

Kleinman, A. (1986) 'Medical anthropology', in A. Kuper and J. Kuper (eds), *The Social Science Encyclopaedia*. London: Routledge and Kegan Paul.

Kushlick, A. et al. (1976) Evidence to the Committee of Inquiry into Mental Handicap Nursing and Care (The Jay Committee), *HCERT Research Report* 129. Winchester: Wessex Regional Health Authority.

Law, J. and Lodge, P. (1984) *Science for Social Scientists*. London: Macmillan. p. 185.

Lewis, G. (1975) *Knowledge of Illness in a Sepik Society: A Study of the Gnau, New Guinea*. London: The Athlone Press.

Lewis, I.M. (1971) *Ecstatic Religion*. Harmondsworth: Penguin Books.

Mann, T. (1960) *The Magic Mountain*. Harmondsworth: Penguin Books. (First published 1924.)

Mauss, M. (1936) 'Les techniques du corps', ounal de psychologie normale et pathologique, 32. Translated in *Economy and Society* (1973) 2(1): 70–88.

Merrison, Sir Alec (1979) *Report of the Royal Commission on the National Health Service* ('The Merrison Report'), Cmnd 7615. London: HMSO.

Murcott, A. (1981) 'On the typification of "bad" patients', in P. Atkinson and C. Heath (eds), *Medical Work: Realities and Routines*. Farnborough: Gower. pp. 128–40.

Ngubane, H. (1977) *Body and Mind in Zulu Medicine: An Ethnography of Health and Disease in Nyuswa-Zulu Thought and Practice*. London: Academic Press. p. 101.

Nuffield Foundation (1986) *Pharmacy*. London.

Oakley, A. (1979) *Becoming a Mother*. Oxford: Martin Robertson.

Oakley, A. (1980) *Women Confined: Towards a Sociology of Childbirth*. Oxford: Martin Robertson.

Rosengren, W.R. and DeVault, S. (1963) 'The sociology of time and space in an obstetric hospital', in E. Freidson (ed.), *The Hospital in Modern Society*. New York: The Free Press of Glencoe. pp. 266–92.

Roth, J.A. (1963) *Timetables: Structuring the Passage of Time in Hospital Treatment and Other Careers*. New York: Bobbs-Merrill.

Roth, J.A. (1977) 'A Yank in the NHS', in A. Davis and G. Horobin (eds), *Medical Encounters: The Experience of Illness and Treatment*. London: Croom Helm. pp. 191–205.

Roth, J.A. and Douglas, D.J. (1983) *No Appointment Necessary*. New York: Irvington.

Sacks, O. (1984) *A Leg to Stand On*. London: Picador.

Savage, W. (1986) *A Savage Enquiry: Who Controls Childbirth*. London: Virago.

Shiloh, A. (1972) 'Equalitarian and Hierarchical patients: An investigation among Hadassach hospital patients', in E. Freidson and J. Lorber (eds), *Medical Men and their Work: A Sociological Reader*. Chicago and New York: Aldine/Atherton. pp. 249–66.

Stacey, M. and Prendergast, S. (1986) Oral contributions to discussion, British Sociological Association Medical Sociology Conference, York.

Strauss, A., Fagerhaugh, S., Suczek, B. and Wiener, C. (1985) *Social Organization of Medical Work*. Chicago: Chicago University Press.

Turner, B.S. (1984) *The Body and Society*. Oxford: Blackwell.

Turner, V.W. (1968) *The Drums of Affliction: A Study of Religious Process among the Ndembu of Zambia*. London: International African Institute, Hutchinson.

Turner, V.W. (1985) 'Images of anti-temporality: An essay in the anthropology of experience', in E.L.B. Turner (ed.), *On the Edge of the Bush: Anthropology as Experience*. Tuscon: University of Arizona Press. (First published (1981) in *Harvard Theological Review*, 75(2): 243–65.)

Turner, V.W. and Turner, E.L.B. (1978) *Image and Pilgrimage in Christian Culture*. Oxford: Blackwell.

Zerubavel, E. (1979) *Patterns of Time in Hospital Life: A Sociological Perspective*. Chicago: Chicago University Press.

Zola, I.K. (1972) 'Medicine as an institution of social control: The medicalizing of society', *Sociological Review*, 20(4): 487–504.

Zola, I.K. (1973) 'Pathways to the doctor – from person to patient', *Social Science and Medicine*, 7: 677–89.

2

Heart Disease and the Cultural Construction of Time

Cecil Helman

For many years, the development of coronary heart disease (CHD) has been known to be associated with a number of 'risk factors' – such as smoking, high blood pressure, raised blood lipids, obesity and diabetes. In 1959, two cardiologists Friedman and Rosenman claimed an important addition to this list which they termed the 'type A' behaviour pattern (TABP) (Friedman and Rosenman, 1959). This was described as a style of overt behaviour, in certain individuals, characterized by the following:

1　An intense, sustained drive to achieve self-selected, but usually poorly defined goals.
2　A profound eagerness to compete.
3　A persistent desire for recognition and advancement.
4　A continuous involvement in 'multiple and diverse functions' constantly subject to deadlines.
5　A tendency to accelerate the rate of many physical and mental functions.
6　An extraordinary mental and physical alertness.

This behaviour was contrasted with a 'type B' behaviour pattern – defined by its relative absence of drive, ambition, competitiveness, sense of urgency, and over-involvement in deadlines. In both cases, diagnosis was initially based on a 'structured interview', where the interviewee's manner and body language were closely observed. If, in the observer's opinion, the interviewee displayed rapid body movements, tense facial and other muscles, 'explosive speech', clenching of hands or teeth, and a general air of impatience – then he or she was classified as displaying the TABP. Later studies added the Jenkins Activity Scale (Jenkins et al. 1979), a 52-item questionnaire, as a more precise tool in diagnosis.

The earliest validations of this classification, in predicting the development of CHD, was the Western collaborative group study (Rosenman et al., 1964, 1975). Over an $8\frac{1}{2}$ year period, 3,154 men aged

39–59 years – all employees of California companies – were initially 'typed' as displaying either type A or B behaviour patterns, and then followed up annually. Of those originally diagnosed as displaying TABP, a significantly higher proportion developed clinical CHD – with a 2.4 times greater risk than those displaying type B behaviour.

Despite the fact that the exact causal link between TABP and the incidence of CHD has not yet been demonstrated (Rosenman, 1978a), and despite several other critiques (Marmot, 1983), this model of pathogenic behaviour has attracted considerable attention, and scores of papers have been written on the subject. Since the 1960s, for example, other authors have widened the definition of TABP beyond the original six core characteristics. By 1983, Burke's review of the subject described type A's 'unbridled ambition', competitiveness, 'free floating hostility', 'high needs for achievement', 'impatience', 'time urgency', and 'polyphasic functioning' (doing many tasks at the same time) (Burke, 1983). Type As also showed greater job involvement, greater identification with the organizations they worked for, and greater 'occupational self-esteem'. Other studies (Burke, 1984) suggested that they were 'work addicts', who had developed a tolerance for work, and who experienced a psychological distress 'akin to withdrawal' if deprived of the opportunity to work. They were particularly attracted to managerial and other high stress careers (Ortega and Pipal, 1984). In academia, type As had higher academic aspirations, were more focused on occupational goals, and often earned higher grades than type Bs (Ovcharchyn et al., 1981); among academic staff, they were more likely to be administrators than professors. Their personal lives were described as emotionally parched and incomplete. They (and their spouses) were less satisfied with their marriages, their jobs had adverse effects on their family and personal lives, they spent little time on leisure pursuits, had few intimate friends, 'rarely savoured joyous moments from the past', were endlessly struggling to enjoy a greater future (which somehow never comes), and generally appeared to have less pleasure and joy in their daily lives than did type Bs (Burke, 1983). Overall, this image of the joyless workaholic, relentlessly on the path of greater wealth, but poorer health, has become a common image in the past 20 years – not only in the cardiology and health education literature, but in popular medical discourse as well.

TABP as a 'cultural disease'

A persistent theme in the TABP literature is that the reasons for the origin, and perpetuation, of this behaviour lie deep within 'modernity' and 'Western culture'. For Friedman and Rosenman (1959) the 'stresses' of contemporary Western life 'are of a variety never pre-

viously witnessed in any previous age of society'. To Rosenman
(1978a), in 1978, CHD was 'the 20th century epidemic', resulting from
'psychosocial factors that are unique to this century'; it is in the
'industrialized 20th century' that the type As struggle to obtain more
and more from their environment 'occurs under repeated stress and
against other persons, things and time itself, leading to a habitual sense
of urgency and an accelerated pace in performing most activities'. In
itself this view of 'modernity' and the (presumed) inevitable 'stress'
that accompanies it, is not new. In 1897 Sir William Osler saw 'arterial
degeneration' as resulting from 'the worry and strain of modern life',
and from 'the high pressure at which men live, and the habit of working
the machine to its maximum capacity' (Osler, 1897). However, the
recent writers on the TABP have added new dimensions to this picture
of a fast, stressful society causing its citizens to lead fast, stressful lives.
Western society is seen as *rewarding* – in terms of money, status,
academic prestige, or control over the environment – this dangerous
form of behaviour. For example, Waldron (1978a, 1978b) explains the
fact that death rates from CHD are twice as high for men as for women
in the United States, as partly due to 'cultural factors' – especially
different American child-rearing practices for boys and girls. Ambition, competitiveness and other type A features are more likely to be
encouraged, and rewarded, in men than in women. Men are expected
to 'succeed in the occupational sphere, whereas women should succeed
in the family sphere; and these two spheres require different behavioural adaptations if success is to be achieved'. For that reason,
TABP is 'more likely to contribute to success in the traditional male
role and much less likely to contribute to success in the traditional
female role'. Therefore, it is more common among employed women
than among housewives (Cohen et al., 1978). Similarly, both CHD and
TABP are less common among non-Western societies, such as the
Japanese. Cohen (1978) ascribes this to their different 'cultural environment' – in particular their emphasis on group rather than in-
dividual achievement, on cooperation rather than competition, and
Marmot and Syme (1976) ascribe increasing rates of CHD among
Japanese immigrants to California as largely due to their increasing
'Westernization'.

Within Western society, some occupational settings are said to
encourage, and reward, TABP more than others: *academia*, as a
setting, 'provides an explicit reward structure that may attract the type
A individual to try to obtain an unlimited number of things from the
environment in the shortest period of time' (Ovcharchyn et al., 1981),
while the *business world* (particularly at managerial level) is characterized by 'a relentless pace, hurried activities, and overload' (Ortega and
Pipal, 1984), and by the 'stressful effects of the rapid social and cultural

mobility found in such settings' (Cohen, 1978). Despite this, type As are apparently attracted to these managerial careers (Ortega and Pipal, 1984); in one study (Howard et al., 1976) of 12 Canadian companies, for example, 61 per cent of the managers were classified as type As. Other studies (Ortega and Pipal, 1984) indicate that in the United States, type As are more likely to be found among managers in rapidly growing firms as opposed to stable or declining firms, in sales or marketing functions rather than accountancy or public sector organizations, and in organizational niches that emphasize the TABP – such as strong orientation to results, as well as time pressure and hard work.

The relationship between the TABP and these social contexts remains controversial (Marmot, 1983). Is the Western milieu the main culprit, and the type A individual the passive victim of its multiple demands? Or does the TABP originate in the individual, as an inbuilt or acquired 'personality trait' or 'behaviour pattern'? Most authors see the TABP as an *interaction* between environmental demands, and a specific 'response style' (Steptoe, 1985) by which certain individuals confront, interpret, and respond to their life situation (Rosenman, 1978b). However, this 'style' of response is frequently described as if it were a more or less static psychological entity – one which has a type of permanence *beyond* these life situations and environmental demands, since it can easily be elicited in the psychological laboratory or interview room, by administering the structured interview or the Jenkins Activity Scale. Hence, in much popular health literature the TABP has been reified to the 'type A personality' (Gibbs, 1979), while in the cardiology literature such individuals are referred to as 'type A individuals' (Ortega and Pipal, 1984), 'type As' (Burke, 1984), 'those with the TABP', 'persons endowed with the TABP' (Byrne and Rosenman, 1986), 'the coronary prone individual' (Gentry, 1978), and those with the 'type A personality trait' (Herman et al., 1986).

Once these individuals have, as it were, acquired the TABP, many of them *choose* lifestyles and occupations consonant with their personal characteristics – organizing their lives in such a way as to expose them to an excess of occupational, social and personal stressors (Byrne and Rosenman, 1986), especially the challenges and competition of managerial (Burke, 1983) or academic (Ovcharchyn et al., 1981) careers.

What then is the origin of this pathogenic behaviour pattern? The predominant approach is to locate its cause within 'Western culture' – in the values, expectations and social organization of industrialization, and 'modernity'. That is, it arises in the very same culture that will one day place such excessive demands on its members, as they grow into adulthood. Price (1983), utilizing a social learning perspective, proposed that personal beliefs or cognitions formed the core of the TABP, and that this behaviour develops to help individuals cope with fears or anxieties associated with certain beliefs they have about the world they live in. These beliefs result from 'socio-cultural values' transmitted to children from their families, schools and mass media of a materialistic society. She identified three beliefs, and accompanying fears, from studies of type A individuals:

1   That positive self-valuation is a function largely of material success, and therefore the individual fears being judged worthless.
2   There are no universal moral principles, and he fears that universal justice and goodness may not prevail ('nice guys finish last').
3   All resources – things worth having – are in limited supply, and life is a 'zero-sum game', and fears he may not get enough of these worthwhile things in his life.

Ambition, too, is learnt from this milieu: according to Rosenman (1978c) extreme type As 'are either born with, learn early, or are parent-trained and instilled with the desire to achieve', while Appels (1973) relates the 'need for achievement' of various cultures to their higher mortality rates from cardiovascular disease. Ovcharchyn and her colleagues (1981) found that type A students reported more parental pressure to attend college than did type B students, and were striving to get jobs concordant with their parents' higher socio-economic status. Socialization into a Western society is therefore held largely responsible, by these researchers, for the development and propagation of the TABP. In that sense, the CHD resulting from this behaviour can be considered – in Appels's (1973) term – a 'cultural disease', closely linked to the 'individual occupational ambitions of Western urban culture' (Steptoe, 1985).

However, some authors have taken this one step further: not only is the type A individual the product, and victim, of modern Western capitalist society – but he is also the *embodiment* (both literally and figuratively) of the values of that society, and of the contradictions between them. For Rosenman (1978c): 'Type A subjects appear to have internalized Western society's emphasis on the ability to master and control their environments'. For Cohen therefore: 'In cultural terms, these men may be seen as overdrawn but accurate images of the Western (particularly American) self-made businessman, living to the fullest the value ideal that you can become anything you desire if you are willing to work hard enough for it' (1978). While for Appels:

> The coronary patient seems to mirror the characteristics of a fast moving, competitive and aggressive society, and, from this point of view, I would like to describe the type A person of Friedman and Rosenman as that person who cannot manage or handle the pressures of the industrialized, fast moving and achievement society and who, by this very failure, shows the characteristics of this society in an excessive way. (1973)

Thus, not only is the type A individual self-destructive, but the cultural values of the society that he comes from are potentially *pathogenic* to large sections of the population – especially if they are middle-aged businessmen. Furthermore, according to Friedman and Rosenman (1971) this risk to health is now increasing, at least in the United States. In their 1960–61 study of over 3,000 male corporate employees in California, approximately half were said to exhibit the TABP, but by 1971 they estimated that 'the incidence in a similar group might approach 75%'. Overall, they estimated then that 'at least 50% of the male population in the large American urban complexes will exhibit the Type A Behaviour Pattern'. Since, as Dressler (1984) indicates, the TABP (and its relationship to CHD) is apparently common in other industrialized societies as well, and as the level of CHD rises with economic development and 'modernization', this phenomenon is of key international concern. Already, cardiovascular diseases are the main cause of death in the United States (Gordon et al., 1974) and in Great Britain (Acheson and Hagard, 1984). If there is, indeed a '20th century epidemic' of CHD, then the TABP is potentially one of the most important public health issues in the modern, in-dustrialized world. As such it deserves closer examination – especially the assertion that it is a Western 'cultural disease'.

To put the TABP model in its cultural context, this paper examines in more detail the following questions:

1   What are the special characteristics of Western cultural *time* – and of the type A's unique relationship to it?
2   What are the *moral* components of this model of a pathogenic society, and its self-destructive citizens?
3   In what sense is the TABP a specifically *Western* – 'cultural disease'? Can it be considered – in anthropological terms – a Western *culture-bound syndrome*?

The nature of Western time

Among the core building blocks of any culture are concepts of space, and concepts of time. Ethnographers have studied differences in the notion of time between societies, and between different populations within these societies. Of relevance here are those studies that have highlighted differences between Western and non-Western time, be-tween industrialized and rural economies.

Hall (1984) has described the predominant form of Western, par-ticularly North American, time as *monochronic*. In this persuasive model, time is seen as linear, as a line or ribbon stretching from past to future, and divided into compartments or segments, such as years, hours, minutes or seconds. Westerners assume that every event or phenomenon will have both a beginning and an end. They also assume that they can only do 'one thing at a time' within each compartment. This linear image is 'woven into the fabric of existence', and co-ordinates everything we do, even moulding our relationships with other people. All social life becomes dominated by schedules and appointments, and thus each conceptual compartment of time seals off one or two people from the wider group, intensifying the relationships between those that exist, temporarily, in the same 'compartment' – while at the same time detaching them from those outside it. For Western people: 'time is an empty container waiting to be filled; furthermore, the container moves along as though on a conveyor belt. If time is wasted, the container on the belt slips by only partially filled and the fact that it is not full is noted' (Hall, 1984).

Each person assumes he or she is the only one who can fill those containers – with productivity, social interactions, or other experiences – and feels he or she 'must make every moment count', lest this tangible time be 'lost' or 'wasted'. To Hall, monochronic cultures are oriented towards 'tasks, schedules and procedures', and thus put a high value on speed and efficiency, on achieving more in less time – as measured by the external standard of the clock. In North America, monochronic time is dominant in the official worlds of business, government, the professions, entertainment and sports. American management, in particular, has over-emphasized monochronic time. Hall sees Western time as unique, in that it originates *outside* the individual; monochronic time, with its segments and schedules, is a form of external *order* imposed on the chaotic lives of humanity. As such – 'Time is organisation'. Scheduling large numbers of people to work or travel at the same time, is an efficient form of social organization; without it, 'it is doubtful that our industrial civilisation could have developed as it has'. In organizations run strictly on monochronic time – such as businesses, schools, hospitals, or the military – this external order is often rigidly enforced, but often at the cost of a 'blindness . . . to the humanity of its members'.

A familiarity with monochronic, clock-time is acquired in almost every Western childhood, reinforced by feeding schedules, school bells, timetables, and an emphasis on punctuality.

What are the origins of this linear conception of time? Needham (1966) sees it as arising from the Judaeo-Christian mythos, with its 'continuous linear redemptive process', which he contrasts with the cyclical, fatalistic time of ancient Greece, Rome and India. For Christianity, linear time was intrinsic, with its progression from the *creatio ex nihilo* to the Second Coming. The world process 'was a divine drama enacted on a single stage, with no repeat performances'. For

Jaques (1982), too, our civilization is characterized by our unconscious 'sense of temporal directionality', reinforced through our
conceptualization of time through spatial metaphors. This linear,
advancing time was, and is, a key feature of Western culture – it
pervaded the ideas of human progress and perfectability of the
eighteenth-century *Philosophes*, the nineteenth-century concepts of
evolutionism, and is still part of contemporary images of 'developing'
nations.

However, monochronic time (like the TABP) is not uniformly
distributed in the Western world, nor is the social organization it
imposes. Hall (1984: 117) sees significant differences between German,
French and American time. Even within the United States, women,
children, the elderly, the unemployed, some ethnic minority communities, and Native American groups such as the Hopi (von Franz,
1978) or the Navaho (Hall, 1984) – all live their lives largely outside
monochronic time. In Japan, also an industrialized society, monochronic time is tempered by traditional Japanese culture; to Nakamura
(1966) Japanese thought 'recognizes absolute significance in the temporary, phenomenal world', and a philosophical willingness to 'accept
the human being's situation in time'. For Hall (1984: 97), in the East,
especially in Zen Buddhism, 'time springs from the self and is not
imposed', in marked contrast to Western time. Within the Western
world, therefore, monochronic or clock-time is one of the organizing
principles of industrialization, but it does not apply to large sections of
the population. It seems to exert its most powerful social force in North
America, among men, especially those working in business or
bureaucracy.

Hall (1984) proposes another, alternative model of time, which
exists in North America and elsewhere. This is *polychronic* time –
which involves doing many things at once, and which stresses involvement of people and completion of transactions, rather than adherence
to preset schedules. For polychronic people, time is not seen as so
tangible or powerful, and punctuality and appointments are not taken
so seriously. Because time is less tangible, it is rarely experienced as
'lost' or 'wasted', and is considered a 'point' (at which relationships or
events converge) rather than a 'ribbon' or 'road'. Polychronic individuals 'are oriented towards people, human relationships, and the
family, which is the core of their existence'; as Hall puts it, 'If you value
people, you must hear them out and cannot cut them off simply
because of a schedule'. In North America, monochronic time dominates the official, public world, but polychronic time takes over in the
home – 'particularly the more traditional home in which women are
the core around which everything revolves'. Hall sees monochronic
time as 'male time', while polychronic time is 'female time', at least

where traditional sex roles exist. The polychronic individual, unlike the clock-dominated person, is involved in multiple tasks, responsibilities, and social ties to other people; time and life are in flux, and nothing is as solid or fixed as the rigidities of clock-time. In Hall's view, polychronic time is also a feature of many non-industrialized societies, as well as some Native American groups.

Not all forms of Western time can be split between monochronic or polychronic forms. Time spent in leisure or contemplation, or in the heightened emotion of ritual or prayer, is qualitatively different from both. Different sections of society – farmers, monks, artists, stockbrokers and executives – all live in different 'time zones', with different relationships to monochronic time. Nevertheless, monochronic time – as measured against the external standard of clocks and watches – is the dominant aspect of Western time. Indeed, one could argue that the *clock*, in all its forms, is the pre-eminent ikon of this civilization.

Time and time-keeping

The rise of time-measurement parallels – and is intimately connected with – the rise of industrial capitalist society. In the early Middle Ages, the cycle of time was linked to religious festivals – Saints' Days, Christmas, Easter, Lent – as well as to the cycle of the seasons, in harvest, mid-summer and autumn festivals. Church bells were among the first time-pieces affecting the life of the population. Mechanical clocks first appeared in European churches and monuments in the thirteenth century (Rawlence, 1985), and were linked to the cycles of prayer. Later, town clocks appeared, which helped regulate the daily work process of its citizens. Clocks owned by individuals, usually only Royalty or the very rich, appeared in Europe in the fourteenth century (Hall, 1984: 129). By the mid-sixteenth century there were established clockmaker guilds in many towns, selling clocks to well-off citizens. In the seventeenth and eighteenth centuries, the notion of a 'universal clock' meting out the one time of the universe, took root. Newton spoke of 'Absolute, True and Mathematic Time' that was universal, and invariable. To Rawlence (1985), this Newtonian–Cartesian thought 'in which clockwork itself had become a metaphor for the nature of the universe', has provided the foundation for the science and technology of today. The new factory system that developed was based on the coordination of large numbers of workers in the same place for the same duration, while the new factory clock (and new technology) imposed a 'dehumanised time discipline' on the workforce, imbuing them with a 'clockwork mentality'. In Britain, by the 1850s, cheaper mass-produced watches were being produced, and there was a huge increase in private watch ownership throughout the nineteenth century

– linking the individual's time permanently to that of the railway timetimes and work schedules of the wider society. By the twentieth century, a monochronic time culture – based on standardized clock-time – was established in most urban centres of the Western world, and watch and clock became familiar ikons of everyday life.

The rise of Western industrial capitalism cannot be explained solely by this spread of clock time. Its roots lie in historical, political, demographic and social factors beyond the scope of this paper. Nevertheless, as Knapp and Garbutt remarked, it is no coincidence that: 'the rise of time measurement as a serious concern, the development of time pieces themselves, the first establishment of time-monitored industrialism occurred in exactly those North European cultures which... fostered entrepreneurship, the rise of capitalism, and strong emphasis upon achievement motivation' (1958).

Clock time facilitated this development by providing an important principle of social organization, that could be imposed from without, control large numbers of people, and increase the speed and efficiency of production. This process required an almost mystical emphasis on *numbers*, on concepts of quantity rather than quality (also a feature of the TABP, Yarnold and Grimm, 1982); a rational organization of time was essential for banking, bookkeeping, and the calculation of interest (Appels, 1982). The units of time had to be quantified, and then linked to units of profit and productivity.

Time as currency

In modern Western culture, time is tangible. It is a multi-vocal symbol, an image that condenses a wide range of meanings. Time is conceived of as a ribbon, a road, a flowing river, as the consumer of man and his works ('Time is all, man is nothing. He is nothing but the carcass of time', wrote Marx (Appels, 1982)) – and as a form of *currency*, or commodity. In popular discourse time can be 'spent', 'invested', 'wasted', 'used', 'bought', 'taken', 'saved', or 'given'; it can be 'free', 'spare', 'extra' or even 'overtime'. Money and goods can be 'bought' with time, and vice versa. In industry, and other aspects of the economy, time, labour, wages, and productivity are all inextricably linked – with the emphasis on producing more, in less time, so as to maximize the margin of profit. In the business world in particular, time is always valuable, and must never be 'wasted'.

For Fraser (1966a) time in the United States has become a commodity, but only present time: 'The past is useless, the Future of interest only as a potentially better present'. What is the origin of this concept of time that must be turned into profit? Weber (1948), in his study of the theological roots of modern capitalism, locates it in the rise of ascetic Protestantism – especially of Puritanism – and its influence on the early settlers of the United States. Early Puritan writers, such as Richard Baxter, preached the virtue of hard, continuous bodily or mental labour, and against 'the spontaneous enjoyment of life and all it had to offer'. Each man's job, or 'calling' was his path to God, if his hard work produced goods for the benefit of the community. 'Private profitableness' was acceptable, provided that its motive was pure – 'you may labour to be rich for God, though not for the flesh and sin'. Wealth was only dangerous when it provided the idleness and leisure that brought with them the temptations of the flesh, and distraction from the religious life. As Weber puts it, to the Puritan:

> waste of time is thus the first and in principle the deadliest of sins. The span of human life is infinitely short and precious to make sure of one's own election. Loss of time through sociability, idle talk, luxury, even more sleep than is necessary, six to at most eight hours, is worthy of absolute moral condemnation...[Time] is infinitely valuable because every hour lost is lost to labour for glory of God. (1948: 157)

By the eighteenth century, both American time and the pursuit of wealth had been stripped of much of their ethical and religious basis: time had become a secular currency. Benjamin Franklin (1794), in his 1736 'Necessary hints to those that would be rich', advised his readers that:

> He that idly loses five shillings worth of time, loses five shillings, and might as prudently throw five shillings into the sea. He that loses five shillings, not only loses that sum, but all the advantages that might be made by turning it in dealing, which by the time that a young man becomes old, will amount to a considerable sum of money.

In modern society, time can be converted to money, and money to time – or rather, to *control* over time. Wealth and status bring the individual power over his own time, and over that of his subordinates, and partial release from the rules of punctuality. Upward social mobility allows the individual, therefore, to break out of the social, economic and time niches to which he has been born.

Quantitative and qualitative time

Implicit in the TABP literature, is the potential conflict between socially imposed clock time, and the psychology and physiology of the individual, that is between quantitative and qualitative time.

This division of public and private, clock and human time is not new. The ancient Greeks differentiated between *chronos* – which Jaques (1982: 14) describes as 'chronological, seriatim time of succession, measurable by clocks or chronometers' – and *kairos*, the 'seasonal time, the time of episodes with a beginning, a middle, and an end, the human and living time of intentions and goals'. In psychological terms, it is the conflict between 'lifeless time' and the 'fused past, present (and future)' of human or living time, between clock time and what Fraser (1966b) terms 'the broad mental present of the subliminal self', ignorant of linear notions of before and after.

Although, in small-scale tribal societies, inner rhythms may mould the pace of daily experience, this is not a feature of urban, industrial life. Obviously, there are circumstances – such as illness, ecstasy, concentration, sex, ritual, dance, or sensory deprivation – where the gap between inner body-mind rhythms and clock time will be very wide. Nevertheless, Western society is unique in trying to impose a fusion between clock time and individual physiology – between rates of bodily movement, speech, gestures, heartbeat, and respiration – and the small machine strapped to the wrist, or hung on the wall. 'Rush hours', deadlines, diaries, appointments and timetables all affect the physiology of modern man, and help construct his world view and sense of identity. *Zeitgebers* – environmental time cues – such as alarm clocks, or the daily roar of early morning traffic, impose their beat on everyday life. In more subtle ways, too, the regular beat of clock time penetrates into human physiology – the contraceptive pill, with its rigid 28-day cycle, being a good example.

Hall (1984: 131) has suggested that in modern society a 'tension' exists between private and public time, resulting in 'stress' and anxiety. For Fraser (1966a), American industrialism, in its rapid pace of development, is in 'a continuous transition, a permanent revolution directed towards a steadily increasing control of the environment', and that this 'anxiety-laden desire for achievement, this holy restlessness en mass' induced a special time-conscious anxiety in those caught up with it.

Although the distributions in the population of monochronic time, TABP and CHD do greatly overlap, there is no evidence that monochronic time directly *causes* the development of TABP. However, there is other evidence of the relationship between imposed social time and damage to health. The calendrical cycle of years, months, weeks, and days has been associated with physiological changes, psychological crises, and increased patterns of pathogenic behaviour – such as the cyclical increase in serum cholesterol in tax accountants in January and mid-April (Friedman and Rosenman, 1971), 'anniversary re-actions' on the same date as a previous bereavement (Musaph, 1973), and increases in violence, alcoholism or suicide on certain religious or public holidays, days of the week. While this may represent a 'tension' in some individuals, between quantitative and qualitative time, these studies do not indicate why some people are affected by clock time, and others are not – a key issue in any discussion of the TABP.

Time and type A behaviour pattern

With this historical and cultural background, the unique relationship of the type A individual to Western, monochronic time can be re-examined. Researchers have suggested that this individual is characterized by a chronic sense of impatience and time urgency (Rosenman, 1978c), is involved with multiple tasks subject to deadlines (Friedman and Rosenman, 1959); tends to accelerate the rate of all his or her activities (such as eating, walking, talking, gesturing) (Rosenman, 1978c); believes that he or she can accomplish more and more in a given time frame, and struggles to do so (Gastdorf, 1980); sets him- or herself high performance standards in terms of quantity, rather than quality (Yarnold and Grimm, 1982); and feels perpetually obstructed by a 'dearth of time' (Rosenman, 1978c). They are excessively punctual and time oriented (ibid.) and in experiments tend to arrive earlier than the type Bs (Gastdorf, 1980), and to work much quicker. In extreme cases, 'he tries to utilize almost every minute of the day in purposeful, goal oriented activity' (Rosenman, 1978c), since everything else is regarded as a 'waste of time'. In the view of Burnham and his colleagues (1975), this time urgency is part of the type A's general coping strategy, aimed at maintaining *control* over his or her social and physical environment, in his or her move towards the ill-defined goal of 'success'. He or she believes that the more problems completed, the more successful he or she is in controlling his or her environment.

Overall, the type A individual is engaged in a 'never-ending struggle with time' (Rosenman, 1978c) – with a struggle 'to overcome the constraints of time' (Burnham, 1975). But what are these constraints against which he or she 'struggles'? The suggestion of this chapter is that these are *social* constraints, and that the clock – as a crucial organizing principle in industrial society – symbolizes control, conformity and cooperation in social and economic life. The type A's struggle to survive and to succeed, occurs against the background of these wider social values – some of which support his or her struggle, while others oppose it – a point discussed below.

Type A behaviour as a culture-bound syndrome

Despite the assertions that TABP (and CHD) is a 'cultural disease' – created and sustained by Western cultural values – a number of problems with the model remain. Firstly, as Rosenman (1978a) himself pointed out, the exact mechanism whereby TABP relates to the incidence of CHD remains to be clarified, especially as CHD has a multi-factorial origin. Other studies (Horowitz and Horowitz, 1986) have been unable to find any clear link between type A behaviour – as identified at interview – and the extent of angiographically determined CHD, nor between this behaviour and subsequent myocardial infarction or coronary death. Furthermore, as Marmot (1983) points out, type A behaviour does not follow the distribution of the population of CHD. For example, in the Framingham study, working women had less heart disease than men, but an equal prevalence of the TABP, while in the Whitehall study, lower income men had a greater risk of CHD, but a lower prevalence of type A behaviour (Marmot, 1983: 382). Therefore, since many of those with the TABP do not develop CHD, and since many of those with proven CHD are not type As, other factors (in addition to TABP) must play a part in the genesis of CHD. A further critique has been that most studies of the link between TABP and CHD have been carried out on 'white, middle-class, middle aged males in the United States' (Cohen et al., 1978), especially those employed in the 'American business world' (Cohen, 1978) – and it is in this community that the link has been most clearly demonstrated, at least in retrospect (Rosenman et al., 1975). Although the TABP, and its apparent link to CHD, has been identified in other Western industrialized societies (Dressler, 1984: 26), many of those cross-national studies have looked at similar (male) populations to the American studies, and of a similar age range (Appels et al., 1982). In some cases, as in The Netherlands, the Jenkins Activity Survey has had to be modified to exclude some questions because of their 'typical American content' (ibid.). In some European studies (Steptoe, 1985), the link between CHD and the TABP has not been found to be as close as in the United States. In the non-Western, non-industrialized world, *no* link has yet been found between CHD and the TABP (Dressler, 1984); for example, a recent study on Kuwaiti Arabs who had suffered a myocardial infarction, found no significant association with previous TABP, and the authors suggested that the TABP might be 'a culture-bound cluster of characteristics' – such as competitiveness and time urgency – neither of which are emphasized in Arab culture (Emara et al., 1986).

Culture-bound syndromes

The inconsistencies in the TABP–CHD model outlined above, lend support to Marmot's (1983) suggestion that 'the measurement and perhaps the concept of Type-A behaviour is not free from culture or class bias'. But how is this cultural bias to be interpreted? The argument of this paper is that, rather than being simply the 'cultural disease' of a pathogenic society, the TABP–CHD model can be considered – in anthropological terms – a Western *culture-bound syndrome*. That is, what is most 'cultural' about this model of the origin of CHD, is the content and boundaries of the model itself.

'Culture-bound syndromes' are specific clusters of symptoms, signs, and behavioural changes recognized by members of a cultural group, and responded to in a particular way. They often link an individual case of ill-health to wider concerns, and have a range of symbolic meanings – moral, social or psychological – for both the victim, and those around him or her. In some cases they play an important part in expressing, and resolving, social conflicts and anti-social emotions, in a culturally-patterned way. In Ritenbaugh's (1982) formulation, they are constellations of symptoms, classified as a 'disease' or 'dysfunction', which are characterized by one or more of the following elements:

1 It cannot be understood apart from its specific cultural or sub-cultural context.
2 The aetiology of the disease summarizes and symbolizes core meanings and behavioural norms of that culture.
3 Diagnosis relies on culture-specific technology as well as ideology.
4 Successful treatment is accomplished only by participants in that culture. Although the symptoms may be recognized, and even similarly organized in other cultures, they are not perceived as the same 'disease' or dysfunction.

In the case of the TABP–CHD explanatory model, the hypothesis developed by cardiologists explains *why* certain people (mainly middle-aged businessmen) in modern industrial society, especially in the United States, develop clinical CHD. The key causal link is between the type A's overt *social behaviour*, and his or her later development of CHD. But a closer look at the constellation of symptoms, signs and behaviours within the TABP–CHD diagnostic category, suggests that their selection is not random – rather, it condenses, and symbolizes, key moral and social concerns of this society.

The model is not, in itself, couched in moral terms. Rather, its imagery resembles that branch of psychosomatic research which, since the Second World War, has ascribed different organic diseases to the specific, pathogenic 'personality type', 'trait', 'profile', 'malfunction', or 'consistent characterological features' of the patient (Helman, 1985). Researchers in this group, such as Alexander et al. (1968) suggested that some organic diseases have not only a specific patho-physiology, but a specific psychopathology as well. Such notions of pathogenic 'personality' or 'trait' can also be understood as deriving from normative models of social behaviour. The emotions or drives associated with these 'personalities' – such as the 'hostility' and 'unbridled ambition' of the TABP – can be seen as cultural constructs, as illustrations of how *not* to think, feel, or act in a particular society. While there is a physiological basis to emotions, they also have a symbolic dimension. Myers (1979) has suggested that the way cultural groups describe 'emotions' can be seen as an ideology, as a model of how one *should* feel and act in relation to others. Emotions that are named and interpreted through socially derived categories (such as 'hostility', 'love', 'fear') represent different types of social relationships, and different relationships of the self to the moral order. In the type A individual, the descriptions of his emotions, drives, personality and behaviour, all imply a 'map' of ideal social values against which he can be measured – a 'map' that applies mainly to Western (particularly American) middle-class, middle-aged businessmen. This model, of how their behaviour leads them to develop CHD, symbolizes – like other culture-bound syndromes – core meanings and behavioural norms of their community, and of the wider society in which they live. The TABP–CHD hypothesis is a model of *morality* – of a conflict between right and wrong behaviour, that must be resolved for the sake of society.

Moral dualism

The moral values implied in the TABP–CHD model are expressed, in much of the literature, as a dualism of type A and type B social behaviour, each associated with the cluster of moral values and other attributes listed in Table 2.1. Although in their original study, Friedman and Rosenman (1959) did include a small third group as

Table 2.1   *Moral values and other attributes of type A and type B behaviours*

Type A	Type B
Hostile	Friendly
Competitive	Non-competitive
Ambitious	Not ambitious
Tense	Relaxed
Greedy	Satisfied
Impatient	Patient
Self-centred	Others-centred
Work-oriented	Family-oriented
Friendless	Friendships
Dissatisfied with socioeconomic status	Satisfied with socioeconomic status
Upwardly mobile	Socially static
Obsessed with time constraints	Indifferent to time constraints
Dangerous to own health	Protective of own health

Table 2.2 *Elements implying moral implication for type A and type B behaviours*

Type A	Type B
Modern	Traditional
Western	Non-Western
Urban	Rural
Fast	Slow
Public	Private
Money	People
Men	Women

control, group 'C', consisting of 46 unemployed blind men, who 'exhibited little ambition, drive or desire to compete', and lived in a 'chronic state of insecurity and anxiety', much of their work dealt with employed men typed as A or B. In a few papers (Appels et al., 1982) a more complex classification was used, including types A1 (the most extreme form), A2 (weak A), A/B (intermediate), B3 (weak B), and B4 (strong B). However, virtually all papers written on this subject have followed the 'binary classification of persons as either Type A or B' (Sparacino, 1979), a fact deplored by recent critics of the model (Horowitz and Horowitz, 1986). This classification is, in effect, a division between values which are socially normative, and those which are *anti*-social – for the opposite of type A values, emotions, and behaviours are those that support the social order of certain groups in society.

Associated with the list in Table 2.1 is another list of elements which regularly cohere in the TABP literature, and which also carry with them moral implication. These are set out in Table 2.2.

From the lists in Tables 2.1. and 2.2, the negative moral qualities of the type A individual become clearer. He is described as a *selfish* individual, who places his or her own interests and advancement over those of family, friends and colleagues. He or she is *hostile* and challenging to work colleagues, always eager to compete with, and rise above them in income and status. By over-zealous behaviours, the type A individual threatens their positions. He or she strives to gain control over his or her time, and presumably over that of others; is *greedy*, and tries to get more time (as currency or commodity) for him- or herself, than he or she would normally be entitled to, that is seeks to do *too much* (including speech, gestures, thoughts, work activities) for the time and social niches allocated to him or her, and which are supported by the organizational principle of clock time. In the struggle to do many things simultaneously the type A individual has, in a sense, polychronic features within the dominance of clock time, but his or her struggle relates to things, not to people.

The TABP is also a *conservative* model of social values, and the type A individual a sort of 'rebel' against the social status quo, though the struggle against constraints is for his or her own benefit, and not for others. Ruthless *ambition* is a key feature of any description of him or her, like the 'keen and ambitious man' described by Osler (1897) in relation to angina sufferers. He or she is *upwardly mobile* (Waldron, 1978b), and dissatisfied with both social status and marriage: work comes before social responsibility to family or friends. The type A's struggle to increase wealth, status, and control over his or her environment is in marked contrast to the type B, whom Rosenman (1978c) describes as 'often very satisfied with his status, both economic and social'. The TABP is also not a feature of the established rich, or of the hopeless poor. Furthermore, women who enter the workforce are more likely than housewives to be classified as type A (Cohen et al., 1978), with all the moral implications of that label. Jenkins's review (1976) of psychosocial factors related to CHD, quotes studies from Sweden showing that women with myocardial infarctions had higher scores on psychological tests for 'aggression', 'achievement', and 'neurotic self-assertiveness', which included 'guilt feelings' and 'defense of status'. If these tests, like the TABP–CHD model, can be considered 'culture-bound', then these diagnostic categories suggest a picture of working women – like type A men – becoming more responsible for their own health, as they become in socioeconomic behaviour more like men.

Furthermore, the type A flouts dominant social mores by the neglect of his or her own health – adopting a 'lifestyle' likely to endanger health, even though aware of its dangers. This contradicts the contemporary ethos, particularly in the United States, which emphasizes self-care and self-reliance in health matters, with jogging, health food and meditation as the pathways to health. Crawford (1977) has argued that contemporary America has greatly reduced the public component of health care, and encouraged people voluntarily to reduce their help-seeking behaviour, and to concentrate instead on improving individual lifestyles, and 'at-risk behaviours'. Much of the current emphasis on at-risk behaviours can be understood as a form of 'victim-blaming' – and, here, the type A individual is the 'victim' to be blamed.

Thus the moral dualism, or competing sets of social values, includes: individual versus group ends, competitiveness versus cooperation, public versus private, work versus home, and business versus domestic ethics. The TABP, therefore, brings danger to more than the individual sufferer. On one level, his or her business behaviour, and the economic system that justifies and rewards it, has a high social cost to less privileged members of his or her society. But the model is less concerned with the macroeconomic system than with the disruptive effects of the type A person's hostility, competitiveness, ambition, greed, selfishness, and over-zealousness on the cohesion and continuity of his work and family networks.

The effect of the TABP on families and friends has been described above (Burke, 1983), but it is just as damaging within a work milieu, for example a corporation. Jay (1972) has described corporations as 'tribes' with their own 'folk culture', traditions, rituals and world-view. Such corporations have rather brittle, unstable hierarchies, since rank and income – at least at the middle management level – are not based on heredity. Competition between businesses, and within them, is part of their ethos, and in a poor economic climate they are subject to sudden fission and defections of personnel. In a phase of shrinking resources, the type A's belief that all things worth having (including time, money and status) are in limited supply, and life is a 'zero-sum game' (Price, 1983) has some basis in reality. Foster's (1965) 'image of limited good' in peasant societies, applies also to the organizations in which the type A works, where all the desirable things are seen as in short supply, so that what one individual gains is at the expense of others. Even in complex, Western societies, wrote Foster 'much of the game of life is played according to the rules of the zero sum' (1972). Therefore, the success of one person breeds envy in the losers, and a sense of guilt in the winner. In his view, envy is bred by the very competitive nature of complex societies, and are a feature of their hierarchical organizations such as government, bureaucracy, corporations, or academia. As one approaches the upper ranks of these organizations, there is less and less room, and the success of one individual prejudices that of those who are competing with him or her. It is in this setting – despite the envy that it provokes – that the type A's struggle to rise in the hierarchy takes place.

Moral ambiguity
Since the TABP is potentially disruptive within small social groupings, it is regarded as a form of *deviance*, as an *over*-conformity with the values of Western capitalist society. More fundamentally, however, the type A individual is a figure of *moral ambiguity* – embodying some of the contradictions in modern social values. His or her behaviour is anti-social, dangerous both to him- or herself and to others, and a threat to the status quo: yet he or she acts in accordance with wider social norms, conforming to what Weber (1948) saw as the predominant ethos of capitalism – 'its philosophy of avarice', and the 'duty of the individual towards the increase of his capital, which is assumed as an end in itself' – and for which he or she is well rewarded. The TABP–CHD model, therefore, suggests a potential contradiction between two sets of moral values – one social, and the other anti-social

– within the same individual. The paradox of the type A individual is that he or she is both social deviant and social conformist at the same time. This paradox suggests that the shift from the puritan image of time as something to be used for the glory of God and the good of the community, to the modern view of time as currency, has been incomplete. Many of the moral imperatives of the puritan ethic survive, in the contemporary image of the TABP.

Resolution of the paradox

The moral paradox in the TABP must be resolved for the good of society, or at least for the good of the individual's social networks. Like other 'culture-bound syndromes', the TABP–CHD model plays a role in expressing, and resolving, social conflict and anti-social emotions. It is a model of human behaviour punished by the development of CHD, and the resolution of the paradox – that anti-social behaviour is rewarded – occurs when the individual actually develops CHD, particularly a myocardial infarction. This resolution takes the form of a 'symbolic inversion'.

Littlewood and Lipsedge (1985) have shown how culture-bound reactions occur 'where major points of political and cultural oppositions are represented in a particular situation', and that these ambiguities or tensions are resolved by the symbolic inversion of social roles. That is, in the course of the reaction, the individual:

> is extruded out of normal social relationships, follows a prescribed role which exaggerates this state, deviant but legitimate, and is then reintroduced into conventional and now unambiguous social relationships ... For the community as a whole, social contradictions are demonstrated but shown to be susceptible of a solution, albeit a temporary and restricted one. (ibid.)

This three-stage process applies also to the type A individual who sustains a heart attack. If the individual survives, he or she too returns to conventional and unambiguous social relationships, chastened, and transformed by the experience in the liminal state of the coronary care unit. During convalescence, and afterwards, he or she is encouraged to be less competitive, ambitious, angry and hostile, less impatient and obsessed with time, and to place more value on home, family, friends, leisure, relaxation, and self-care. In short, the individual is encouraged to convert from type A to type B. The process is thus:

$$\text{Type A} \rightarrow \text{Myocardial infarction} \rightarrow \text{Type B.}$$

The individual also becomes more 'female', in terms of traditional, stereotyped roles, and less of a 'super-male'.

By becoming, at least temporarily, a type B, the ambiguity and contradictions inherent in the TABP model are largely resolved. This resolution by inversion of roles strengthens, and reasserts, the social values of the social networks in which the type A is embedded. Deviance is punished, and the status quo reasserted; the deviant is reintegrated into family and firm, chastened, fragile, dependent, and less competitive.

Type A in popular culture

The cardiologists' etic models of the TABP, and its link to CHD, summarize and symbolize core cultural meanings and behavioural norms for middle-aged men in Western society. The techniques of diagnosis – the structured interview and the Jenkins Activity Survey – can, like other social science research, also be considered 'culture-bound'. Indeed Rosenman (1978c) has admitted that the interview method 'is an empirical instrument that is not truly objective'. However, these etic models do not exist in isolation: biomedical models of disease have increasingly diffused into popular culture, often in a distorted form. References to 'the type A personality', and the role of 'lifestyle' in coronary heart disease, are common in radio and television programmes, newspapers, magazines, home doctor books, and other self-help literature. Unlike much of the cardiology literature, the emphasis is less on the pathogenic role of Western society, and more on the individual's responsibility for his or her own ill-health. In this emic model, the 'type A personality' has entered the canon of impure behaviour, that marks the victim of CHD from the rest of society. The way that popular culture constructs the TABP and its consequences, also makes it a culture-bound syndrome. Both lay and medical models can only be understood in their specific context, in the ways that they express key concerns of Western, industrial society, particularly in the United States.

The dangers of impatience and haste have long been noted in popular folklore, for example in proverbs such as 'Haste is from the Devil', 'Haste trips over its own heels', or 'Haste makes waste'. Today the image of the 'hasty person' appears in much of the 'stress' and 'lifestyle' literature. Recent books on stress reduction echo the binary classification of 'personality types' into types A and B (Rudinger, 1982), while those on lifestyle and CHD often include descriptions of the type A's 'coronary-prone behaviour', 'hurry sickness' and 'time urgency' (Gibbs, 1979). A patient advice pamphlet *Recovering from your heart attack* advises:

> The dangerous stress is that which the individual brings on himself, not that which is imposed by others. Aggressive, competitive individuals who are over time-conscious, and find it difficult to relax have a far higher risk of suffering a heart attack than more passive non-competitive people. Try to learn to relax – forget about deadlines. Stop competing and start to delegate responsibilities. (Pharmax, undated)

While a book on 'time management' (Lakein, 1973) with chapters on 'Making the Most Out of One Spare Minute', 'Make Your Sleep Work for You', nevertheless warns about becoming a 'compulsive clockwatcher', like the 'time nut'. This 'notorious character' is 'overwhelmingly preoccupied with time. He makes himself and everyone else nervous with his concern about never wasting a minute. He's always rushing around to meet an impossible schedule . . . Not an easy person to work or live with.'

Whether described as 'type A personality', 'hurry sickness' or the 'time nut', lay images of the TABP mirror those of the cardiologists, but with more emphasis on the individual's culpability for his or her own ill-health. In a study of the health beliefs of 150 managers of medium and large corporations (Albrecht et al., 1982), heart disease was placed high on their list of stigmatized conditions, as persons with heart disease were considered especially responsible for their conditions. In Cowie's (1976) study, patients recovering from a myocardial infarction in a coronary care unit, engaged in retrospective reconstructions of their own biographies, in such a way that their heart attack was perceived as the obvious outcome of their previous lifestyle – a point of view shared with other patients and with medical staff. This image of the heart attack as nemesis, has also been noted by Cassell (1976) among his patients. According to him, heart attacks in the United States have acquired their own 'mythology': 'We even feel that we know who is going to get one. "If he keeps on going like that", we say, "he's going to have a heart attack." In our minds, heart attacks have a relationship to what we do, as though we bring them upon ourselves.'

Conclusions

The argument of this chapter has been that the TABP, and its suggested link with CHD, can be considered a Western culture-bound syndrome, mainly involving middle-aged, middle-class, North American businessmen. It cannot be understood apart from its specific cultural and historical context, since it symbolizes core concerns and social norms of Western society. Diagnosis relies on culture-specific ideology and technology, and successful treatment can only be achieved by members of this society. It also links individual cases of ill-health to wider concerns, and carries a range of symbolic meanings for both the victim and those around him or her. Finally, it can play an important role in resolving ambiguities and tensions within certain social relationships.

Seeing the TABP–CHD model as essentially 'culture-bound' does not make it in any sense less true or real. Nor does it diminish its obvious value in epidemiological research, or in predicting or preventing CHD. But it does acknowledge that diagnoses such as 'type A behaviour' or 'coronary heart disease' have moral components unique to our culture, and that these may influence clinician and patient alike.

References

The article contained in this chapter first appeared in *Social Science and Medicine*, 25, 1987.

Acheson, R.M. and Hagard, S. (1984) *Health, Society and Medicine*. Oxford: Blackwell. p. 58.

Albrecht, G.L., Walker, V. and Levy, J. (1982) 'Social distance from the stigmatized: a test of two theories', *Social Science and Medicine*, 16: 1319–27.

Alexander, F., French, T.M. and Pollock, G.H. (eds) (1968) *Psychosomatic Specificity*, vol. 1. Chicago: University of Chicago Press.

Appels, A. (1973) 'Coronary heart disease as a cultural disease', *Psychotherapeutics and Psychosomatics*, 22: 320–4.

Appels, A. (1982) 'Cultural aspects of coronary prone behavior', *Advances in Cardiology*, 29: 32–6.

Appels, A., Jenkins, C.D. and Rosenman, R.H. (1982) 'Coronary-prone behavior in The Netherlands: a cross-cultural validation study', *Journal of Behavioral Medicine*, 5: 83–90.

Babcock, B.A. (ed.) (1978) *The Reversible World: Symbolic Inversion in Art and Society*. Ithaca, New York: Cornell University Press.

Burke, R.J. (1983) 'Career orientations of type A individuals', *Psychological Reports*, 53: 979–89.

Burke, R.J. (1984) 'Beliefs and fears underlying type A behavior', *Psychological Reports*, 54: 655–62.

Burnham, M.A., Pennebaker, J.W. and Glass, D.C. (1975) 'Time consciousness achievement striving, and the type A coronary-prone behavior pattern', *Journal of Abnormal Psychology*, 84: 76–9.

Byrne, D.G. and Rosenman, R.H. (1986) 'The type A behaviour pattern as a precursor to stressful life-events: a confluence of coronary risks', *British Journal of Medical Psychology*, 59: 75–82.

Cassell, E.J. (1976) *The Healer's Art*. Philadelphia: Lippincott. pp. 41–2.

Cohen, J.B. (1978) 'The influence of culture on coronary-prone behavior', in T.H. Dembrowski et al. (eds), *Coronary-Prone Behavior*. New York: Springer. pp. 191–8.

Cohen, J.B., Matthews, K.A. and Waldron, I. (1978) 'Coronary-prone behavior: development and cultural considerations', in T.H. Dembrowski et al. (eds), *Coronary-Prone Behavior*. New York: Springer. pp. 184–90.

Cowie, B. (1976) 'The cardiac patient's perception of his heart attack', *Social Science and Medicine*, 10: 87–96.

Crawford, R. (1977) 'You are dangerous to your health: the ideology and politics of victim blaming', *International Journal of Health Services*, 7: 663–80.

Dressler, W.W. (1984) 'Social and cultural influences in cardio-vascular disease: a review', *Transcultural Psychiatric Research Review*, 21: 5–42.

Emara, M.K., Fakhr El-Islam, M., Abu Dagga, S.I. and Moussa, M.A. (1986) 'Type A behavior in Arab patients with myocardial infarction', *Journal of Psychosomatic Research*, 30: 553–8.

Foster, G.M. (1965) 'Peasant society and the image of limited good', *American Anthropology*, 67: 293–315.

54   Time, health and medicine

Foster, G.M. (1972) 'The anatomy of envy: a study in symbolic behavior', *Current Anthropology*, 13: 165–202.

Franklin, B. (1794) 'Necessary hints to those that would be rich', in *Works of the late Doctor Benjamin Franklin*. London: Robinson. pp. 60–5.

Fraser, J.T. (1966a) 'Comments on time, process, and achievement', in J.T. Fraser (ed.), *The Voices of Time*. London: Allen Lane. pp. 136–9.

Fraser, J.T. (1966b) 'The study of time', in J.T. Fraser (ed.), *The Voices of Time*. London: Allen Lane. pp. 582–94.

Friedman, M. and Rosenman, R.H. (1959) 'Association of specific behavior pattern with blood and cardiovascular findings', *Journal of the American Medical Association*, 169: 1286–96.

Friedman, M. and Rosenman, R.H. (1971) 'Type A behavior pattern: its association with coronary heart disease', *Annals of Clinical Research*, 3: 300–12.

Gastdorf, J.W. (1980) 'Time urgency of the type A behavior pattern', *Journal of Consulting and Clinical Psychology*, 48: 229.

Gentry, W.D. (1978) 'Behavior modification of the coronary-prone behavior pattern', in T.H. Dembrowski et al. (eds), *Coronary-Prone Behavior*. New York: Springer. pp. 225–9.

Gibbs, R. (1979) *Lifestyle and Coronary Heart Disease*. London: Macmillan. pp. 55–68.

Gordon, T., Garcia-Palmieri, M.R., Kagan, A. et al. (1974) 'Differences in coronary heart disease in Framingham, Honolulu, and Puerto Rico', *Journal of Chronic Diseases*, 27: 329–44.

Hall, E.T. (1984) *The Dance of Life: The Other Dimension of Time*. New York: Anchor Press.

Helman, C.G. (1985) 'Psyche, soma and society: the social construction of psycho-somatic disorders', *Culture, Medicine and Psychiatry*, 9: 1–26.

Herman, S., Blumenthal, J.A., Haney, T., Williams, R.B. and Barefoot, J. (1986) 'Type As who think they are type Bs: discrepancies between self-ratings and interview ratings of the type A (coronary-prone) behaviour pattern', *British Journal of Medical Psychology*, 59: 83–8.

Horowitz, R.I. and Horowitz, S.M. (1986) 'The coronary-prone behavior pattern', *Archives of Internal Medicine*, 146: 1429–32.

Howard, J.H., Cunningham, D.A. and Rechnitzer, P.A. (1976) 'Health patterns associated with type A behaviour: a managerial population', *Journal of Human Stress*, 2: 24–31.

Jacques, E. (1982) *The Forms of Time*. London: Heinemann.

Jay, A. (1972) *Corporation Man*. London: Jonathan Cape.

Jenkins, C.D. (1976) 'Recent evidence supporting psychologic and social risk factors for coronary disease', *New England Journal of Medicine*, 294: 1033–8.

Jenkins, C.D., Zyzanski, S.J. and Rosenman, R.H. (1979) *Jenkins Activity Survey Manual*. New York: Psychological Corporation.

Knapp, R.H. and Garbutt, J.T. (1958) 'Time imagery and the achievement motive', *Journal of Personality*, 26: 426–34.

Lakein, A. (1973) *How to Get Control of Your Time and Your Life*. New York: Signet p. 15. p. 15.

Littlewood, R. and Lipsedge, M. (1985) 'Culture-bound syndromes', in K. Granville-Grossman (ed.), *Recent Advances in Clinical Psychiatry*. London: Churchill Livingstone. pp. 105–42.

Marmot, M.G. (1983) 'Stress, social and cultural variations in heart disease', *Journal of Psychosomatic Research*, 27: 377–84.

Marmot, M.G. and Syme, S.L. (1976) 'Acculturation and coronary heart disease in

Japanese Americans', *American Journal of Epidemiology*, 104: 225–47.

Musaph, H. (1973) 'Anniversary disease', *Psychotherapeutics and Psychosomatics*, 22: 325–33.

Myers, F.R. (1979) 'Emotions and the self: a theory of personhood and political order among Pintupi Aborigines', *Ethos*, 7: 342–70.

Nakamura, H. (1966) 'Time and Indian and Japanese thought', in J.T. Fraser (ed.) *The Voices of Time*. London: Allen Lane. pp. 77–91.

Needham, J. (1966) 'Time and knowledge in China and the West', in J.T. Fraser (ed.), *The Voices of Time*. London: Allen Lane. pp. 92–135.

Ortega, D.F. and Pipal, J.E. (1984) 'Challenge seeking and the type A coronary-prone behavior pattern', *Journal of Personality and Social Psychology*, 46: 1328–34.

Osler, Sir W. (1897) *Lectures on Angina Pectoris and Allied States*. New York: Appleton.

Ovcharchyn, C.A., Johnson, H.H. and Petzel, T.P. (1981) 'Type A behavior, academic aspirations, and academic success', *Journal of Personality*, 49: 248–56.

Pharmax Ltd (undated) *Recovering from Your Heart Attack*. London.

Price, V.A. (1983) *Type A Behavior Pattern: A Model for Research and Practice*. New York: Academic Press.

Rawlence, C. (1985) 'Clock time', in C. Rawlence (ed.), *About Time*. London: Cape. pp. 32–58.

Ritenbaugh, C. (1982) 'Obesity as a culture-bound syndrome', *Culture, Medicine and Psychiatry*, 6: 347–61.

Rosenman, R.H. (1978a) 'Role of type A behaviour pattern in the pathogenesis of ischaemic heart disease and modification for prevention', *Advances in Cardiology*, 25: 35–46.

Rosenman, R.H. (1978b) 'Introduction', in T.H. Dembrowski et al. (eds), *Coronary-Prone Behavior*. New York: Springer. pp. XIII–XVI.

Rosenman, R.H. (1978c) 'The interview method of assessment of the coronary-prone behavior pattern', in T.H. Dembrowski et al. (eds), *Coronary-Prone Behavior*. New York: Springer. pp. 55–69.

Rosenman, R.H., Brand, R.J., Jenkins, D., Friedman, M., Strauss, R. and Wurm, M. (1975) 'Coronary heart disease in the Western Collaborative Group Study: final follow-up experience of $8\frac{1}{2}$ years', *Journal of the American Medical Association*, 233: 872–977.

Rosenman, R.H., Friedman, M., Straus, R., Wurm, M., Kositchek, R., Hahn, W. and Wethessen, N.T. (1964) 'A predictive study of coronary heart disease: the Western Collaborative Group Study', *Journal of the American Medical Association*, 189: 15–22.

Rudinger, E. (ed.) (1982) *Living with Stress*. London: Consumers Association. pp. 68–9.

Sparacino, J. (1979) 'The type A (coronary-prone) behavior pattern, aging and mortality', *Journal of the American Geriatrics Society*, 27: 251–7.

Steptoe, A. (1985) 'Coronary-prone behavior', *British Journal of Hospital Medicine*, 33: 257–60.

Von Franz, M.-L. (1978) *Time: Rhythm and Repose*. London: Thames & Hudson. p. 5.

Waldron, I. (1978a) 'Type A behavior pattern and coronary heart disease in men and women', *Social Science and Medicine*, 12B: 167–70.

Waldron, I. (1978b) 'Sex differences in the coronary-prone behavior pattern', in T.H. Dembrowski et al. (eds), *Coronary-Prone Behavior*. New York: Springer. pp. 199–205.

Weber, M. (1948) *The Protestant Ethic and the Spirit of Capitalism*. London: Allen & Unwin.

Yarnold, P.R. and Grimm, L.G. (1982) 'Time urgency among coronary-prone individuals', *Journal of Abnormal Psychology*, 91: 175–7.

3

Time and the Cervix

Hilary Thomas

In the social and cultural construction of the events of a woman's reproductive and sexual anatomy and in the medical speciality of obstetrics and gynaecology time is literally 'of the essence'. It is fundamental to the constitution, organization and interpretation of symptoms, and to the delineation of the normal, the abnormal and the pathological. As Richman and Goldthorp observed: 'in the consultation, mutual concern about time, in its multifaceted guises, becomes a domain activity which operates as both a topic of enquiry and a resource for developing explanations to achieve a provisional resolution of the often conflicting demands and beliefs of patient and gynaecologist' (1977: 160).

Frankenberg has argued that biomedicine is distinguished from other healing systems by the bounded, asymmetric and contradictory temporalities of its practitioners and their patients. Time is essential in the control of transitions between the hospitalized body and the embodied patient. He concluded: 'The contradiction of temporalities and of aspects of body boundaries is sharpest between social and natural motherhood on the one side and class and gender-constructed obstetric medicine on the other' (Frankenberg, 1988: 31).

Pizzini (1992), in an exploration of aspects of the clash of temporalities within the labour ward, observed, importantly, that practitioner time could not be simply equated with objective time since an important subjective element entered practitioners' use of time.

Differences and disjunctures are not confined to the clash between lay and medical perspectives for, as Emily Martin has recently written: 'What all women in our society share is the experience of housekeeping of their own bodies, whose effluvia, demands and exigencies so seldom appear in schedule with socially organised time' (1989: 201).

Much of the temporal interest focuses on the cervix, the pivotal point for the uterus and the gateway between uterus and vagina. And, as any gateway, it must be open(ed) or closed as and when appropriate. Much obstetric interest in the cervix is concerned with the control of access between the two areas, and in particular medicine's ability to control access. Quite a variety of substances pass, or fail to pass, through the cervix in the course of their lawful, or unlawful, business. Time, then, becomes the means by which ordered and orderly transitions can be identified.

This chapter focuses on temporal aspects of passage through the cervix in three areas: menstruation, conception and in pregnancy and its outcomes. Comparison is made between women's and medicine's use of time and relative control over temporal aspects of these areas. Speculation about the relationships between degree of control and the location of that control in time itself are offered in conclusion.

The fate of the uterine lining

The uterine lining may be transformed into the normal products of menstruation and make an orderly transition. Conversely that transition may be too rapid or too frequent for the comfort of the woman, and this may be seen by her doctors as having some underlying pathological cause. The onset and cessation (be it permanent or temporary) of such transitions accompany important status passages, for example, in menarche, pregnancy and menopause. Time is inextricably bound up in such transitions.

Menarche indicates the imminent onset of fertility. In contemporary Britain, while it is not usually marked by overt ritual its arrival will frequently have social meanings beyond the potential for childbearing. Preparation for menstruation in the form of knowledge leads to an expectation that it should occur. If a girl knows that other girls have started having periods she may interpret the non-arrival of her own as an indication of abnormality: '[When I started] I was quite pleased, really, that I was normal, because I was so much later than all my friends were ...'.[1]

The proper time to start periods is therefore socially situated and may lead to a sense of injustice:

> I considered myself a late starter and it frightened me because I didn't think I was going to have one. 'Cos my sister – she's younger than me – and she'd started, you see. And I used to say to my mother, 'Oh, it's not fair: she has and I haven't and I'm older than her!' [and my mother would say] 'It's not your age it's your size,' but I didn't understand that at the time.

Having periods may confer status as part of an 'in' group. Conversely being among the first to begin could be fraught with other meanings: 'It was something I wasn't expecting I suppose. I'd been prepared for it but I suppose it did come as a bit of a shock ... I felt a bit of a freak 'cos I was only 11.'

The primary notion of time in menstruation is of course the regularity and frequency of the cycle, notions which are themselves imbued with cultural connotations. To have a 28-day cycle is not only to have a regular cycle but it is to have *the* regular cycle. Thus regular cycles of other lengths may be described as 'irregular' and may be regarded as a deviation from the norm. One of the actions of the combined oral contraceptive pill is to establish a 28-day cycle. This may be seen as an advantage. It may also be seen as an interference with the natural processes of a woman's body. Literally speaking, of course, it is, but the particular imposition of a different cycle and alterations in the volume and velocity of menstruation, may cause concern.

What the pill also provides is the opportunity to reschedule menstruation:

> The pill certainly eased the flow off considerably and of course it makes it so much more sort of sociable, really that you can confine it to a certain time period and if it isn't convenient for you then you can mess about with your pills as you like, really, if it's going to involve a holiday or something you can delay it....

Missing a period or 'being late' raises the possibility of pregnancy during the earlier years of a woman's fertility. Later this may be interpreted as a feature of the menopause.

More frequent bleeding than usual may lead to tiredness and a feeling of being drained. It may also cause the woman to seek help from a doctor to alleviate the speed of transition or to exclude the possibility of some pathological condition. The circumstances in which the unusual becomes the unbearable may be directly related to the context of everyday activities. Thus a woman who had heavy periods and had recently been moved to work in a sealed unit said:

> [it has] finally come to the crunch – I've got to wear all-in-one white overalls with just a bra and pants underneath and that creates all sorts of problems... I work in a sealed production unit where we have to change our clothes to go through the different stages of our work, therefore we've got communal changing rooms and if I've got three or four pads on with the likelihood of bleeding further then it's going to be a problem – it's just going to come through onto the white overalls – and once we're in the sealed units we can't come out for so long, you know, ... I'm in there for an hour or two hours... Before I was working in the [other] unit where I could pad myself up and it, it wasn't quite so bad. But now I'm beginning to get a bit desperate. Because if it happens there I've got a problem, you know!

She went on to explain that this was particularly difficult since most of the people she worked with were 'young chaps straight from university'. The meaning of menstruation had changed for her not only because of the change in her working environment, but because of her own gynaecological history. She had always had heavy periods, though they had become worse. However, in the past she put up with these because she was undergoing infertility investigations in order to try for a second child. As she explained, heavy periods, regular periods were a good sign for the prospect of pregnancy. She had several infertility investigations which were accompanied by a D&C operation[2] to try to 'calm' the periods. Her wish to get pregnant preconcluded other forms of treatment:

> I think when you're trying – I think it's all psychological, really – when you're trying to have a baby it rules your life and everything else gets pushed into the background. I think always our prime, or my prime reason for going to see the doctor in those years . . . was to get pregnant, and if I had to put up with very heavy periods then I'd put up with them, you see, at that stage they didn't want to give me any form of medication in case I did get pregnant . . . It's only since we've decided that that's finished, we won't try anymore, that I've been doing – also they've got worse – but I've been more constructive about getting some treatment.

Alterations in the speed of transitions can be interpreted by a woman in terms of her obstetric and gynaecological history, as in the train of events experienced by a woman who noticed heavier bleeding after her third Caesarean section. She was also sterilized at the time of the third section and attributed the dramatic blood loss in hospital to the fact of the sterilization. When her periods returned they were also heavy and she assumed that this was also due to the sterilization. Fear of a hysterectomy kept her from the GP for over a year, until desperation with the bleeding exceeded her anxiety. Her GP diagnosed fibroids, later confirmed by a D&C, and explained that these could be caused by the Caesarean incisions. The woman, while accepting the diagnosis still felt that the proximity to the sterilization must account for some of her trouble.

A number of different kinds of time are invoked by the perception and meanings of menstruation. Richman and Goldthorp observed:

> The gynaecologist often has difficulties in deciphering whether a patient's opening description of a symptom, especially of a repetitive bodily function of a period, . . . as opposed to something 'new' or 'different', can be classified as medically abnormal. The patterning of the activities can be differently associated with, for example, aging and can still be normal clinically. 'Lengthy' periods, 'irregular' periods, 'painful' periods, 'heavy' periods, 'short' periods, 'missed' periods can, in given contexts, be regarded as medically appropriate. (1977: 169)

Attribution of meaning does not change only for the gynaecologist. How a woman copes with menstruation may depend on the context in which it occurs. The context can be the time schedule of the workplace in which breaks which permit use of the toilet may be timed by the work process rather than by biological time. Extended leisure time may be experienced as inappropriate time for menstruation and oral contraception may be used to reschedule this. The same rate of flow may be perceived by a woman as desirable or undesirable as her fertility aspirations change. Similarly irregular periods may be perceived as usual for a particular woman until reclassified as a sign of possible fertility problems. Changes in the pattern of menstruation may be located as disorder of the body in terms of time arrangements, and may then raise issues of pathology. Such changes may be located by the woman within the sequencing of her own reproductive and body history. Onset and cessation of menstruation are situated both within the time stages of the individual life-course and in relation to peers. Menstruation may thus be out of time for the 8-year old or the 80-year old, for the youngest middle school pupils or the members of a retirement club.

Time and conception

Eggs and sperm make various kinds of transition through the cervix. Only sperm make the vagina-to-uterus passage as unaccompanied minors; eggs are released into the uterus as part of treatment for infertility, though given the amount of paraphernalia this process requires the egg could scarcely be described as being unaccompanied. Both make the reverse journey as separate, unentwined, reproductively functionless entities. It is the task of barrier contraception to prevent live sperm from reaching the cervix; part of the action of the combined oral contraceptive pill is to produce a plug of mucus which deters sperm. In infertility treatment part of the diagnostic procedures involve attempts to ascertain whether sufficient sperm have survived to reach the cervix.

The time and timing of conception and birth are, of course, bound up with pre- and proscriptions, not least of which are those concerning maternal age usually expressed in terms of chronological years but incorporating both social age and biological age. Conception is expected to be planned. Planned pregnancy implies not only a wanted child but a timed child. Family planning implies not only limitation of the total number of children but the timing and spacing of births. At the antenatal clinic a woman who has planned a birth by desisting from oral contraception may find that she still fails to meet the exacting standards of medical and midwifery staff whose concern to calculate the date of delivery may be thwarted by the woman's menstrual history. It is not enough to stop contraception because a baby is wanted, but rather 'proper' periods must be resumed before any attempt is made to conceive. It is not unusual for women to report that they have been 'told off' at the antenatal clinic for trying for a baby immediately after oral contraception instead of employing a barrier method. What is being timed here is conception, not birth.

It seems that most couples in Britain plan their families and employ contraception in order to achieve their wishes (Dunnell, 1979). What began as an attempt to time births to avoid maternal exhaustion (Leathard, 1978) – a reference to cultural interpretations of physiologic time – has become transformed into other meanings of time. Women report that they wish to avoid having children too close together because the work involved in attending to one small baby is made more difficult by the addition of a second child. But also there are reports that each child should have time for him- or herself without competition from a younger sibling.

The concept of family planning itself not only implies a metaphor of housekeeping but is inextricably bound up with its skills, namely the constant fight against disorder, be this of a financial, temporal, spatial or emotional nature. Having too many children or too few, having them too close together or too far apart, is thought to entail, variously the risks of hardship, indulgence, untidiness, loneliness or neglect. A 'proper' family can be recognized by a well-ordered house(hold). The middle class view of the converse was well described by Rosamond Lehmann in a novel first published in 1932. She described the sweep's family of eight:

> Regularly once a year the new baby became the old baby. There seemed no warning, but there it was – another weevil, blanched, shrivelled, perfectly silent, carried forth from the cottage triumphantly among them for an airing as ants convey an egg. Each year you didn't think they'd rear it, but they did. Tough as stonecrop it pushed up, and joined the others on the railings. They were the worst family in the neighbourhood. Their cottage was unwashed, unswept, littered with broken glass, broken china, odds and ends of soap-box and bedding: a dreadful problem. (1932/1981: 74)

Use of contraception within the family planning process stands at the juncture of two temporal spheres. First, family planning aims to place the existence of a baby in the household at a preferred time within the life-course. It should be noted that the right 'time' to have a baby may be perceived in general terms of chronological age (not 'too young', not 'too old') but may also be measured in terms of acquisition of suitable housing, steady employment and a certain amount of material possessions. Second, especially for those women who have used oral contraception, contraceptive practice is supposed to incorporate timing of the birth, to facilitate a more precise anticipation of date of delivery and hence assist with the medical enterprise of pregnancy in terms of measurement of gestation and surveillance of foetal development. Thus 'proper' use of contraception incorporates aspects of the time worlds on either side of the hospital boundary.

The issue of control is more problematic for contraceptive use than for menstruation. Failure to prevent unintended pregnancies may occasionally be seen as the result of contraceptive failure, sometimes as the result of inappropriately-delivered services, often as the result of failure of the couple and usually as the failure of women to ensure adequate protection regardless of inadequate methods, services and partners.

Pregnancy and its outcomes

It seems probable that most pregnancies are lost, that they pass through the cervix unknown to the woman either as unimplanted or dislodged embryos (Oakley et al., 1984). In termination of pregnancy it is a temporal measure of gestation in terms of weeks which indicates when this might be performed, in addition to consideration of the other circumstances of the woman and the pregnancy, and of which surgical method should be employed.

In the continuing pregnancy gestational time is used to determine the pattern of antenatal care and to provide evidence of the health and well-being of the foetus. The pattern of antenatal vists is itself a temporal sequence whose intensity increases with advancing gestation. Thus, 'monthly visits to 28 weeks, fortnightly to 36 weeks and weekly thereafter' is a form frequently quoted, though less often strictly adhered to (Thomas et al., 1983), that it seems surprising to learn that its origin is nothing more grand than a Memorandum from the Ministry of Health, issued in 1929 (Oakley, 1986: 79). Attempts to renegotiate the structure based on an appraisal of the efficiency of antenatal care have not met with widespread acclaim (Hall et al., 1980). Such timing may not suit a woman's own identification of her needs. A woman who has miscarried early during a previous pregnancy may be surprised that there are not rather more visits at a similar time during her current pregnancy.

Rather little can be done by way of intervention during pregnancy apart from delivering the baby prematurely. Most effort goes into surveillance rather than management, and is a form of fact-gathering for the time when the baby will be delivered. Estimation of the date of delivery is thus a primary function of midwifery and obstetrics. Birth thus becomes not 'her time', to use a biblical phrase, but 'their time'. In particular 'their time' is calculated using 'their methods'. It is no longer enough to keep note of menstrual dates, though, as we have seen, failure to do so may lead to a reprimand from staff concerned. Rather the full impact of modern technology is brought to bear in the form of ultrasound technology. This enables staff not only to predict the future but, in some sense to see it, in the form of the image on the screen. What is measured is the foetus and therein lies the first of numerous translations of time into other calibrations.[3] The dimensions of foetuses are thought to be sufficiently similar during the second trimester that gestation can be calculated from measurement of the size of the foetus.

Graham and Oakley (1981) point out that use of ultrasound provides a technique which increases and supports medical rather than maternal expertise. This linking of time and size conflicts with what is self-evident to women: that all babies are different. As one woman said: 'They seem to go by averages too much so they measure the head and know how many weeks you are. So they are saying that all babies are the same size!' (Draper et al., 1984: 138).

The certainty with which the ultrasound gestation is invested can cause considerable anxiety for a woman who is equally certain about her own information about gestation. One woman wrote the following in answer to a question about whether anything had worried her about the scan: 'Being told my dates must be wrong since the baby was so small. Had to return for second scan. I knew my dates were right therefore I was worried about my baby being small' (ibid.: 134).

Antenatal care provides a lot of information about the health of the baby and the likely outcome at birth. In addition to size, where 'small for dates' and 'large for dates' babies cause concern, movement is thought to be an indicator of well-being. The development of foetal movement charts, on which a woman is asked to note the time at which the baby has kicked ten times during the day, are thought to secure information about appropriate movement during pregnancy, particularly towards the end of pregnancy (Pearson and Weaver, 1976). If the baby has not achieved ten kicks within the allotted twelve hours, the woman is advised to contact a practitioner for guidance. What such a system does not allow for are babies who are active outside that time period: 'I was a bit confused because there was so much variation from day to day. Naturally I was worried. I would rather not have filled it in as my baby was more active at night time' (Draper et al. 1984: 120).

At the end of gestation lies birth, the timing and progress of which have been major sources of discord between women and their birth attendants (Cartwright, 1979; Oakley, 1980; Graham and Oakley, 1981). It is not merely the fixing of the estimated date of delivery which causes such problems, but the course to be followed once such a date is reached. Induction of birth not only shifts delivery into an approved gestational sequence but allows for the birth itself to be managed within staffing time schedules: confinement confined. And within the extension of 'her time' to whose time is the baby itself:

> they weren't sure of my dates but the first doctor give me the 4th of October and she stuck to it, but the [hospital] doctor kept putting it a month later because of my periods not being what they wanted it to be . . . Well, actually I went into labour on the 4th of October and they wouldn't let me have him.

They stopped him – put up drips and things and stopped him, said that he was a small baby, so they held him off a fortnight . . . they didn't think he was ready. Well, obviously he must've been ready or else he wouldn't've wanted to be born.

During a continuing pregnancy vaginal examinations are performed to check the condition of the cervix for the foetus must be retained during pregnancy but expelled during parturition. A cervix which cannot retain the foetus – an 'incompetent' cervix in obstetric discourse – may be stitched. During parturition, in addition to the timing of contractions, the cervix gives evidence of the progress of labour. It must open at a given speed – one centimetre per hour – until completely dilated. The failure to dilate either at the correct speed or at all has contributed to the development of techniques of induction and acceleration during hospital birth.

In a woman who has not borne a child the cervix is described as being 'untried' and therefore it is not known whether it will prove fit or incapable during birth. A woman whose cervix has been tried – usually taken to be delivery after 28 weeks of pregnancy – is regarded in obstetric terms as parous. But the cervix also has a special role in the demarcation of the stages of labour and delivery. The first stage is completed by the full dilation of the cervix, the next stage the delivery of the baby, the third stage being delivery of the placenta. During parturition, then, it is the negotiation of the cervix by the baby which turns a labour into a delivery, a pregnancy into a birth and a pregnant into a parous woman.

In pregnancy and birth the baby moves through various stages of potentiality to the child in the present. In miscarriage and stillbirth matter is not only out of place (Douglas, 1966/1984) but out of time (Allatt, 1992). It is out of time in three senses. First there may be a premature delivery, a gestation ended too soon. Second, and more mysteriously, the child of the future moves into the past within the biography of the parents. Third, the customary ordering of events which holds that life precedes death and that birth precedes dying, has become confused. A child who dies before it is born presents a shocking challenge to that temporal order. It may be that when the parents of a stillborn child describe holding the dead baby as a positive experience (Lovell, 1983), that one of the things which this action does is to create the sense of a present and an existence, if not life, for that child within that present. In miscarriage the experience may be more difficult to comprehend since the sense of the pregnancy may have been constituted as a feeling of sickness or of imagination with no bodily changes. Lewis (1985) describes these events as the black magical events of reproduction, and talks of the woman who gives birth to the stillborn baby as delivering into the grave.

Properly, then, birth precedes death, and in particular a baby's birth properly precedes the mother's death. In contemporary medicine the death of the mother may hasten but not always determine the demise of the child since technology may be employed to provide support mechanisms essential for the maintenance of placental function after brain death in the mother has been established.

During pregnancy relatively little can be achieved except refinement of measurement of the foetus, measurement which always stands in some relation to gestation, a medical perspective of pregnancy time. This is both to establish a precise time date for the birth and to record the development of the foetus to establish the size of the baby that will be delivered. Intervention in the continuing pregnancy is limited to measures to prevent spontaneous premature delivery and occasionally to induce premature delivery of a baby that is failing to thrive in the uterus. In contrast, both labour and delivery are rich in potential for medical midwifery intervention, in particular for temporal change and control. Medicine appears to have least to offer in the circumstances of maximum temporal disruption attendant upon stillbirth. It has also been slow to recognize that miscarriage at an earlier stage of pregnancy may also entail a deep sense of loss and require appropriate expression of grief.

Conclusion

In matters of reproduction, time appears in a variety of forms and serves an assortment of purposes. It is employed in its different forms by the various parties interested in the events of reproduction. Thus any understanding of time must identify which time and whose time is involved. The complexity of the derivation of any particular temporal sequence, meaning, or interpretation is increased by the transformation of time into other measurements. Thus gestation becomes size and weight. The cervix is the site of many of the transformation scenes of reproduction: in acting as gatekeeper, medicine finds its role to be that of timekeeper.[4]

Time provides not only a way of describing the distribution of events but also a basis for interpretations and explanations. In reproduction it provides a way of distinguishing between normal and the abnormal, between the abnormal and the pathological. More generally this can be seen as a differentiation of the ordered from the disordered, the orderly from the disorderly.

With the exception of menstrual extraction by vacuum suction little control can be exerted by either the woman or medical personnel over the speed of passage of the uterine lining through the cervix at that time. Possible control must be exercised prior to actual menstruation by drugs, or by the diagnostic surgical procedure of D&C which has a temporary efficacious effect in some women. Such control is largely located within medical frameworks of reference. Oral contraception, which requires a prescription, does however have the potential for rescheduling of menstruation by women themselves. In conception and its counterpart control over passage through the cervix may be exercised close to the time of intercourse if barrier methods are used. What have been seen as theoretically more reliable methods of preventing pregnancy, such as the pill, the IUD or sterilization, must be employed further away in time. The greater opportunities for medical control over negotiation of the cervix, during birth, are employed close to the time of passage: coeval control.

Notes

1. This paper draws on data produced in several studies undertaken by the author concerning contraception, antenatal care and gynaecological surgery. (Quotations are referenced where they have appeared in published work.)

2. Dilatation and Curettage (D&C) is a commonly performed gynaecological procedure in which the cervix is dilated and the contents of the uterus removed.

3. I am grateful to Ronnie Frankenberg for this observation.

4. Again, I am grateful to Ronnie Frankenberg for this observation.

References

Allatt, P. (1922) *Time and Dis-ease* (Chapter 9, this volume).

Cartwright, A. (1979) *The Dignity of Labour*. London: Tavistock.

Douglas, M. (1966/1984) *Purity and Danger: an analysis of the concepts of pollution and taboo*. London: Ark Paperbacks.

Draper, J., Field, S. and Thomas, H. (1984) *An Evaluation of a Community Antenatal Clinic*, Occasional Report. Cambridge: Hughes Hall.

Dunnell, K. (1979) *Family Formation 1976*. London: HMSO.

Frankenberg, R. (1988) ' "Your time or mine?" An Anthropological View of the Tragic Temporal Contradictions of Biomedical Practice', *International Journal of Health Services*, 18(1): 11–33. (See also Chapter 1, this volume.)

Graham, H. and Oakley, A. (1981) 'Medical and maternal perspectives on pregnancy', in H. Roberts (ed.), *Women, Health and Reproduction*. London: Routledge and Kegan Paul.

Hall, M., Ching, P.K. and Macgillivray, I. (1980) 'Is routine antenatal care worthwhile?', *Lancet*, 12 July: 78–80.

Leathard, A. (1978) *The Fight for Family Planning*. London: Macmillan.

Lehmann, R. (1932/1981) *Invitation to the Waltz*. London: Virago.

Lewis, E. (1985) Paper to the Royal Society of Medicine Forum on Maternity Care and the Newborn, London.

Lovell, A. (1983) 'Some Questions of Identity: Late Miscarriage, Stillbirth and Perinatal Loss', *Social Science and Medicine*, 17(11): 755–61.

Martin, E. (1989) *The Woman in the Body*. Milton Keynes: Open University Press.

Oakley, A. (1980) *Women Confined: Towards a Sociology of Childbirth*. Oxford: Martin Robertson.

Oakley, A. (1986) *The Captured Womb*. Oxford: Blackwell.

Oakley, A., McPherson, A. and Roberts, H. (1984) *Miscarriage*. London: Fontana.

Pearson, J.E. and Weaver, J.B. (1976) 'Fetal Activity and Fetal Well-being: An Evaluation', *British Medical Journal*, 277(i): 1305–7.

Pizzini, F. (1992) 'Women's Time, Institutional Time' (trans. by R. Frankenberg), (Chapter 4, this volume).

Richman, J. and Goldthorp, W.O. (1977) 'When Was Your Last Period? Temporal Aspects of Gynaecological Diagnosis', in R. Dingwall et al. (eds) *Health Care and Health Knowledge*, London: Croom Helm.

Thomas, H., Draper, J., Field, S. and Hare, M.J. (1983) 'An Evaluation of the Practice of Shared Antenatal Care', *Journal of Obstetrics and Gynaecology*, 3(3): 157–60.

4

Women's Time, Institutional Time

Franca Pizzini

Anyone who thinks about time in relation to pregnancy and childbirth will realize that they raise many fascinating questions. Above all a distinction has to be made between physiological or body time, psychological time or time of the mind, and social time pertaining to society, each with their own characteristics, rhythms and rules. Should one also distinguish pregnancy time and childbirth time?

The time feeling which seems to me closest to that of pregnancy (thinking both of my own and that of the many women to whom I have spoken) was time of the unconscious or the time of involuntary memory which we associate with Proust. (I don't think it was merely chance which led me to reading *Remembrance of Things Past* during my first pregnancy or that my daughter is called Albertina.) Unconscious time is that which emerges unbidden from involuntary memory, and which is made up of recollections, fantasy, dream and reality. A memory which emerges only at specific moments when the Narrator in the Proustian context (the woman-narrator or protagonist) can let himself go to listen to his own interior world. But his 'letting oneself go' requires a social justification: for her arising from her status as pregnant woman, for him (the Narrator of *Remembrance*) from his status as a man touched by art, to whom 'revelation' permits the transformation of life into art, days into works. This literary comparison, however, refers also to the traditional image of relations between the sexes: woman completes her work through a child, man through art and culture. I certainly do not wish to give credence to such an image when I refer to the universality of a writer who has intuitively suggested themes utilizable in a 'feminine' way in relation to a matter so distant to him as pregnancy.

The question that follows from this evocation of Proust is necessary to my theme: is there an unconscious time, an interior time as opposed to a social time-in-the-world? Many women's experience in pregnancy shows not only that there is, but that this time of listening inside is closely related to body time. Many women tell of their own pregnancy that it was a time of fullness, of joy and of satisfaction, arising more from the state itself than from the expectation of a child. They speak of a 'suspended' time in which they have been 'empowered' socially and legitimately to live their own status without external worldly obligations. This is an experience of today's women, in whom the unconscious is expressed in a different way from that of women of epochs when pregnancy was more often necessary than desired, when work (in field or factory) could not be given up and for whom a domestic fate was the only one possible.

In the accounts of women interviewed, it was often said that giving birth came like the rupture of an equilibrium, like an event which turned upside down the former state of well-being. What is this feeling due to? To the fact that giving birth is in any case an upsetting event through which women pass to become two, to put an end to symbiosis and to begin separateness? Or to the fact that physiological time, body time changes to a more socially defined time through the medium of the people that attend her? I think the various elements play their part in combination with one another.

There is already in the historical memory of women the fact that giving birth represents a moment of rupture, a life crisis, during which the woman must be accompanied by persons who in her specific culture are designated for such a function. In traditional societies there were wise women (mammane) or birthing companions (comari), then licensed midwives and finally doctors. The person who traditionally attended the woman in labour was someone who came to her house, to her own territory at the beginning of labour, and the attendance continued throughout the birth and the early postnatal period. The place was the same as that where the pregnancy had been lived through, the break therefore was one of time only not of place: that meant (and means still for those who are able to have that experience) that the break came to be seen as less violent.

Women who give birth these days generally live through an experience of break between the inside and the outside (home and hospital) which can have repercussions within their own internal world. They thus pass from the daily domesticity of their own pregnancy to being hospitalized with the beginning of labour. Such a transition means above all that the time in which the individual woman has become immersed becomes a time which is substantially institutional, socially determined. The logic of the many prevails over the logic of the individual.

This can be shown by an example which we have found again and again in our researches on the maternity hospital (Colombo et al., 1985). The woman in labour with contractions coming at certain regular intervals is taken into hospital; immediately the pains cease and only restart later when the woman has accustomed herself to the change of place, or else after a medical pharmacological intervention to restart them. Women verbalize the experience of hospitalization as central. They recall it as a moment which represents a break with the entire lived process up to then: they talk to the hospital personnel referring persistently to a 'before' at home and an 'after' which means 'after being taken into hospital'. We can therefore say that hospital childbirth is an experiential break, as much historically as in the life of individual women and that giving birth at home has a very progressive aspect in such experience.

Let us now look at how the theme of time has always been very relevant both for those giving birth and for those who attended them. The months and days of pregnancy are counted and noticed as are the hours of labour and the moment of giving birth: even after years women remember most of these details in a very precise manner. They say, for example, 'For my first child, it took me twelve hours, for the second, nine'; 'He was born at six-fifteen after six hours of labour'; 'The contractions began at four o'clock'; 'Between one contraction and the next there was five minutes at first'; and so on.

Traditionally, in fact, the signs connected with the progress of pregnancy and of birth came to be read on the body of the woman, came together to be interpreted by her asking herself about her own feelings. When pregnancy and birth were medicalized, the signs came to be read by machines, on the monitor, through chemical reactions and through microscopes. That which the woman senses or lives is no longer important; indeed often what she explains or relates comes to be seen by the technician-doctor as embarrassing or confusing the objective tests of science. Such a scientific definition demands that the individual timing of each specific pregnancy ought to correspond as nearly as possible to predictable rules and to codified factors. So that if a woman does not begin labour at the expected time, after the given number of weeks according to medical statistics, doctors intervene to promote labour through pharmaceutical induction. No account is taken of subjective diversity through which some delay could have been caused by physiological, psychological or social factors, but the process is rationalized, reducing it to an experience which takes account only of medical competence. The woman may believe that this type of intervention is necessary for her own health and that of her child, but at the same time may also recognize the violence being done and the doubtful utility of its application to each single case. It depends on what kind of woman she is and what attitude she has to medicalization.

Is it possible for us to say that there is one time for the childbearing woman and another for those who are supposed to be helping her? This has certainly become true with the movement of childbirth into the hospital. The distinction between the two perceptions is accentuated giving rise to a real dichotomy between personal, physiological individual time and institutional time. Let us now look more closely at the workings of the institution of maternity to give some examples to confirm what we have been asserting. It is perhaps useful to go back to the article on 'The sociology of time and space in the obstetric hospital' by Rosengren and DeVault (1963).

They carried out their research by prolonged observation within a maternity hospital. They argue that they were increasingly impressed by the fact that the behaviour of personnel seemed to differ markedly depending on where it took place and in what sequence. 'The structures of both time and space appeared more and more to serve to delineate status and define roles' which made evident 'the notion of the importance of the physical setting'. This led them to focus still more on what they saw and heard 'more specifically in terms of time and space associations' (ibid.).

I believe, as far as space is concerned, that our researchers have gone beyond Rosengren and DeVault, because we used a more complex construction and more precise observations derived above all from Goffman (1969) and Hall (1966) as well as various studies in social geography (Pizzini, 1985). As far as time is concerned it still seemed to us interesting to use the distinctions in their article between, first, rhythm, second, time and third, timing (coordination and synchronization between rhythm and time) and I give here some examples from our researches.

The rhythm of activities: the periodicity at which events happen (When?)

This periodicity is contingent and depends on the type of patient with whom staff find themselves confronted. For example, if the woman giving birth is considered to be a 'bad patient', someone who does not fit in with expectations from the viewpoint of the staff, she receives quite different treatment from someone considered to be 'good'. She is visited less, but also, if she cries out and gets agitated, receives more medical interventions aiming to get the event over and done with. Things which are described by health workers as medical necessity, immutable procedures in time and in space, are in fact changed according to variations between the people involved in the interaction. For example a midwife about to finish her shift and go home, can speed up the rhythm of intervention by carrying out an amniorexis (rupturing the membranes) at a different moment to that provided for by the hospital administration, let us say at a dilatation of 2–3 cm instead of at one of 6–7 cms.

Time: timing, the number of interventions which happen during a unit of time (How many?)

This refers to the number of births which take place in a given period of time and in relation to the time of the institution. In 24 hours there could be two or three or fifteen to twenty: this lack of a naturally based tempo would seem (as it did to Rosengren and DeVault) to be made use of in many different ways, which are not so much related to 'physiological' as to 'functional' time. For example, when two births are happening a short distance apart, the staff become very anxious, and continuously check the signs of progress in labour. Thus an excessively prolonged labour upsets the medical team just as much as does a precipitate birth, re-emphasizing the strictly defined conception of normality on which the institution of maternity is based. The 'normal, correct' time for a birth is defined by a subtle, equilibrating, interplay between physiological processes, medical intervention, professional skill and the reactions of the woman giving birth to such intervention. Each hospital has its own implicit norm (often not recognized by those who operate it) which defines the time duration of labour and birth acceptable to the staff. Often physiological time hardly enters into such schemes, hence interventions which are particularly useful at keeping time within the limits considered to be normal: forceps in the United States, Caesarean section in Italy. Such practices are often considered acceptable even in situations where the only pathology is that the duration of the process is considered to be excessive.

Timing: coordination and synchronization between rhythm and time (In what relationship?)

Temporal institutional organization is able to take place through the sequences of 'timing': the woman in labour's trajectory through medical procedures is scrupulously followed by the staff even when it is not necessary, in such a way that all procedures are completed in due order and at established times. Sometimes 'physiological time' would require leaving one or more procedures or stages in the trajectory of the woman giving birth, but she has to adapt herself to this predecided rhythm even when for her it presents a useless struggle. For example, a woman bearing her third child was about to give birth so precipitately that there was no time to complete the 'prep-procedures' which were however carried out just the same. The obstetric team were very agitated lest the baby was born before this and the father was sent home being told that it was a case of 'false contractions'. These kinds of deviation from 'timing' are upsetting for the staff, but timing and rhythm of procedures are not in fact immutable if the changes are made by the staff itself. For example, there is a very great difference in the behaviour of doctors on night duty and those on days: at night-time some procedures are not practised, even if during the day they are considered essential. For example, sampling amniotic fluid which is discoloured would indicate the immediate necessity of Caesarean section happens much less in the afternoon than in the morning, when the operating theatre is in full swing. It also happens more in the daytime when the full staff is on duty rather than at night. Similarly, oxytocin drips to accelerate labour are not set up at night although during the daytime they are a routine procedure for all women in labour. Such facts throw doubt on the very idea of 'medical necessity' declared to be beyond discussion by obstetric rationality.

A final example on this aspect concerns the perception by staff of how long different phases of giving birth should last. For example, we calculated that in the final stage of actual delivery, staff perception was at least double the reality: the staff who attended the woman in the delivery room recalled a final period of one hour whereas in fact it lasted a half of that. They claimed also to have left the baby with its mother immediately after birth for at least ten to fifteen minutes, when in fact according to our calculations, this period was never longer than five minutes.

This paper began by reporting our initial observations on the dichotomization between subjective and objective time; evidently this division does not only exist for the woman in labour but also for the staff who attend her. We have observed that rhythm, time and timing assume greater importance as one gets nearer to the delivery room itself, often a separate space from the ward where the rest of labour has taken place. Rosengren and DeVault also noted as we did that this transition is marked by a speeding up of gesture and movement, an increase in the number of staff present and a kind of frenzy of activity which involves the whole situation. This speeding up is understandable, if one thinks of the moment of birth as the culmination of a long process, perceived by those who assist in it as strongly and emotionally involving, even when medical rationalization seeks to schematize and routinize it to hold in check its disruptive force. In our culture this is further legitimated by the greater presence of doctors in the delivery room compared with earlier zones of the maternity hospital. In the preparation rooms and the general labour wards, midwives and nurses on their own are more often present than doctors.

In traditional cultures the number and kind of persons present is substantially the same for the whole process of labour and birth. The hospital division of labour has on the other hand parcelled up the process, dividing times, spaces, persons present according to the particular procedure being carried out on the woman giving birth. This corresponds to a division of her body into areas of interest: we have called that from the waist to the head 'affective' and that below 'technical', which represents the field of work of the staff. Such a division is related more to the organization of the hospital than to the physiological and psychological rhythms of the woman giving birth. The relationship between these two times raises the problem if not of mediation between them at least of establishing an equilibrium which would not be totally out of the control of the woman giving birth, something which has not happened as yet in many hospitals despite years of reflection, of struggles, critiques and proposals for change.

Notes

This chapter was translated by Ronald Frankenberg.

References

Colombo, F., Pizzini, F. and Regalia, A. (eds) (1985) *Mettere al Mondo: La produzione sociale del parto*. Milan: Franco Angeli.

Goffman, E. (1969) *Strategic Interaction*. Philadelphia: University of Pennsylvania Press.

Hall, E.T. (1966) *The Hidden Dimension*. New York: Doubleday.

Pizzini, F. (1985) 'Note sullo spazio nel reparto di maternita' in G. Colombo, F. Pizzini and A. Regalia (eds), *Mettere al Mondo: La produzione sociale del parto*. Milan: Franco Angeli.

Pizzini, F. (1989) 'The expectant mother as patient: a research study in Italian maternity wards', *Health Promotion*, 6(1).

Rosengren, W.R. and DeVault, S. (1963) 'The sociology of time and space in an obstetric hospital, in E. Freidson (ed.) *The Hospital in Modern Society*. New York: The Free Press of Glencoe. pp. 266–92.

5
Doctors, Patients and Time

Peter Pritchard

Time, along with space and energy are major dimensions of living and working, yet time in general practice has not been studied in any depth. But ask general practitioners what their main problem is, and most will answer 'lack of time' (Donald, 1985). Similarly, when patients are asked about general practice, frequent complaints are about time – that the consultation is too short and that the doctor is hurried (Social Research Unit, NOP Market Research, 1982).

General practice is a major part of the British National Health Service (NHS), responding to about 80 per cent of episodes of illness and providing the first point of access to other services. In the United Kingdom, general practitioners (GPs) have a list of patients for whom they are responsible, today typically about 2,000 patients per doctor, who on average see their GP about four times a year. The time spent in each consultation averages 5.5 to 8.25 minutes (Bradley, 1983; Wilkin et al., 1986; DHSS, 1987), compared to Finland and Sweden where the normal booking time is 20–30 minutes. Dr John Horder, a former President of the Royal College of General Practitioners, has called this short consultation time a national disgrace (Donald, 1985).

These timings are not immutable. Recent studies in London have shown that when the booking rate was lowered from one patient every 5 minutes to one every 7.5 or 10 minutes, measurable benefits followed, such as more problems being identified, patients' and doctors' satisfaction increased, blood pressure recorded more often, more explanation given and prevention discussed (Morrell et al., 1986).

Clearly, UK GPs have a problem with time, but what is less clear is the nature of the problem and whether any remedies are possible. The main aim of this chapter is to explore the temporal issues facing general practitioners and patients in order to seek practical ways of improving the effectiveness of primary health care. The chapter is set out in five main sections: general practitioners and time; time for patients; the doctor's time apart from patients; kinds of time in general practice; and practical action for GPs.

A number of themes run through all the sections. One is the difference between taking a short-term and a long-term view – of the doctor's work, of the patient's illness and of the interaction between doctor and patient in the context of illness. Another theme is whose time it is, and this ownership of time is bound up with issues of power and potential conflict. There is also the theme of time as an independent variable constructing social reality, like the seasons; or as a dependent variable constructed by events, some of which we may be able to influence, for example, work schedules or timetables. The final theme is the flow of understanding about time across boundaries of knowledge and discipline, and the impact that this might have on the care of patients.

General practitioners and time

How general practitioners spend their time
There have been several international surveys on how much time doctors spend consulting with patients. Hull (1983) for instance, has shown that GPs in Canada headed the list, with an average of 5.75 hours a day spent consulting and half an hour visiting, whereas GPs in the United Kingdom were bottom of the list with 3 hours on average spent in consultation and 1.33 hours visiting. In Sweden 4 hours consulting and 0.75 hour visiting were reported. Hull also showed that GPs in the United Kingdom typically worked a 10 hour day as follows: 4 hours consulting; 1.5 hours home visiting; 1.5 hours doing hospital and other outside work; 2 hours learning and teaching; and 1 hour on administration and medical politics.

A more recent British government survey of GPs' self-reported workloads (DHSS, 1987), showed that contracted NHS 'general medical service duties' averaged 38 hours per week, but 15 per cent of GPs worked over 50 hours and 12 per cent less than 25 hours per week. Other duties, outside the NHS contract, occupied 6 hours per week, and in addition GPs were on call for an average of 30 hours per week. This made a total working week of 44 hours, with a further 26 hours a week on call. Again the variances were large, with 12 per cent of GPs working more than 110 hours and 11 per cent less than 35 hours per week (excluding time on call); 87 per cent of the duties were between 8.00 am and 7.00 pm (weekdays) and 8.00 am and 1.00 pm (Saturdays).

Interestingly, those doctors who had the services of more employed and attached staff, such as secretaries, practice nurses, health visitors and district nurses, worked relatively longer hours, but presumably the content of their work was different. Time spent on call may be inactive, but many doctors cannot relax when they are on call at home and find it stressful for themselves and their families. The boundary between work and non-work is blurred and being called out becomes intrusive.

Where (as in Finland) time on call is usually spent at the health centre, the boundary is clearer but there is no evidence that the strain on the doctor and family is any less.

Trends in workload (Fry, 1983) have shown a doubling of night calls (11.00 pm to 7.00 am) between 1967 and 1976. Between 1969 and 1979 surgery consultations increased by 7 per cent, home visits decreased by 41 per cent, and other services, such as telephoning, dictating letters and meetings, increased by 250 per cent. Total face-to-face meetings between doctors and patients (a sum of consultations and visits) had decreased by 4.5 per cent. These surveys have all relied on GPs' own reports of how they spent time, rather than external observations.

A longer view of general practitioners' time
General practitioners tend to settle in a permanent post early in their career, and so would have the opportunity for long-term planning. However, personal experience has indicated that GPs are not keen on planning ahead. Once settled in a locality, their work goes on unchanged with no promotion or advancement except to senior partner. Many GPs find it monotonous to see 30 to 40 patients a day year in and year out until they retire, particularly those GPs who think that many of their patients' reasons for attendance are trivial.

Other GPs take a broader view of their role in the community and find great satisfaction in the interpersonal contacts and the long-term relationships with families and the local community. There seems to be a link between GPs' view of the frequency of 'trivia' in consultations and their long-term job satisfaction and perception of their standing in the community (Cartwright, 1967). The same study by Ann Cartwright showed that the GPs with a high 'trivia' score were less likely to attend postgraduate courses or have access to hospital beds. The discrepancy between the value that doctors set on their time and the way patients use a doctor's time, may account for some of the labelling as trivia.

Some GPs counter this lack of satisfaction in their everyday work by undertaking medical work outside the practice such as hospital, school or factory sessions, or they can become a GP-teacher, or take part in administrative work. These parallel activities all compete for the doctor's time, the loser often being time for the family. The family may take second place to a demanding and open-ended job until retirement or death.

Traditionally, the male general practitioner's wife may be so tied to the practice and the telephone that an independent career is difficult. Women general practitioners are now being trained in equal numbers, so the temporal structure and social organization of general practice will need to change.

General practice: doctor-led or demand-led?
Demand for service in the British NHS mostly operates through the practice organization. Some demand goes direct to the doctor when on call at night, or meeting patients in the street. Doctors are partly in the organization, and partly isolated in the consulting room or doing home visits.

When doctors perceive that the workload is excessive, they can put up barriers to demand – lengthen the waiting time for appointments; stop sessions at strict times; maintain a high booking rate; or seem to be in a hurry – all building up the belief that the doctor's time is more valuable than the patient's, and that patients are a nuisance. Posters may appear in the waiting room with a very negative message: 'Don't bother the doctor if you can help it'; 'Ring before 10 if you need a visit'; and so on. Patients may start to wonder if they even have any right to be ill.

Is time a problem for general practitioners?
Most caring professions see time as a problem and articles about occupational stress and 'burnout' abound (Jones, 1981; Porter et al., 1985). Huntington (1981) has suggested that GPs' time orientations differ from those of other occupational groups in the health care system on account of their preoccupation with pressure of time. General practitioners, when questioned about the nature of their time problems, emphasize five main features: the unpredictability of demand; the heavy and apparently increasing workload; the lack of structure of their time; their lack of ability to organize their time effectively; and finally their personal difficulties in coping with conflicting calls on their time, leading often to workaholism or alcoholism.

These replies are symptomatic of a disorder of time management. To use a medical metaphor – the symptoms can be treated one by one at a superficial level, or an attempt can be made to understand the underlying nature of the time problems (the physiology and pathology), before making a diagnosis and applying treatment.

Time for patients

What patients feel about time in the context of general practice
Two linked surveys, in 1964 (Cartwright, 1967) and 1977 (Cartwright and Anderson, 1981), showed that patients' perceptions of time problems had worsened in the 13 years separating them, as shown in Table 5.1. This apparent worsening of patient satisfaction may have arisen partly out of GPs' insensitivity to patients' feelings and needs, and partly from a rise in patients' expectations. Whatever the explanation,

Table 5.1 *Proportion of patients who felt their doctor was 'not so good' about various aspects of practice*

	1964 %	1977 %
Always visiting when asked	3	13
Keeping people waiting in the waiting room	17	21
Taking time and not hurrying you	6	14
Explaining things fully to you	16	23

Sources: Cartwright, 1967; Cartwright and Anderson, 1981.

there is no cause for pride. Dissatisfaction with the time GPs spend with their patients was greater among those who had psychological problems, people who did not know the doctor and the young (Cartwright and Anderson, 1981). Another study has shown that 'rushing patients or being abrupt' were seen as by far the most unsatisfactory characteristics of the GPs studied. This was remarked on by 33 per cent of respondents, as compared with only 11 per cent who thought that the GP was incompetent (Arber and Sawyer, 1979).

When patients were asked informally, such as in a patient participation group (Pritchard, 1986) what sort of time problems they perceived, the following points were made:

1 Doctors were seen as busy people whose time should not be wasted.
2 Consultations were often delayed until the problem became very urgent because patients were anxious about 'bothering the doctor' for trivia.
3 Visiting the doctor upset routine and placed the patient under time-pressure from outside (for example, work, family commitments).
4 Being ill can distort time (because of anxiety or pain), and extra time was needed to cope with illness or disability.
5 Getting to see the doctor took time – time to get through on the phone, past the receptionist, the delay of waiting for an appointment and then in the waiting room.
6 Consultation time was experienced as too short for tackling the problem adequately.
7 Doctors were seen as unsympathetic and uncaring about other demands on the patient's time such as family commitments.

When a patient consults a doctor it is the start of a continuing process – a trajectory of sickness. The GP, however, may just see each visit as an episode separated in time from other events – like one snapshot in a pile of hundreds. The interaction could be likened to a moving train. The patient (in the train) observes an unfolding landscape from starting point to destination. The GP (on the platform) sees a series of windows flashing by, and has to try to put together a coherent view of what is going on behind all those windows. From a snapshot of the present, the GP has to link past events and current data in order to predict the likely course and outcome of the disease. Patients may find it difficult to understand that the doctors do not have the same biographical view of the illness as they do – or in the case of a strange doctor who has not read the notes – no biographical view at all.

The GP's time is broken up into small segments, described as 'fractured time' (Huntington, personal communication). This is at odds with the need to reflect from longer-term experiences.

Continuity of care over a longer time-scale
Personal doctoring and continuity of care are often quoted as important ingredients of general practice (Gray, 1979), but not everyone seems to be convinced. Surveys of patients suggest that they rate 'seeing the same doctor' very highly. From the doctor's viewpoint, continuity of care may mean, at best, looking after individual registered patients, particularly those with chronic disorders, for a working life of around 30 years, apart from holidays and off-duty periods.

Even if the general practitioner stays in the same locality, the population moves around. So the span of continuing care might cover childhood and childbearing, or from middle age until death, but never 'from cradle to grave', except for a very few with short life spans. Any beliefs that doctors may have that they are providing lifelong care is an illusion, based on a composite of people or a succession of doctors in a practice.

What is the extent of continuity when a general practitioner retires or dies? Is there an overlap period with the succeeding doctor? This is unlikely if the senior doctor is taken ill and does not return. More often now, the succeeding doctor is an ex-trainee who has been working in the practice for a year, which makes for good induction. If practices in the United Kingdom did pursue a policy of overlap, they would have to accept a loss of income.

The patient's medical record is another vehicle for continuity, though it tends to be impersonal, and to concentrate on the technical details rather than on the sum of biographical details that makes up the patient's identity. The essence of continuity of care is that the patient's identity is preserved intact and that the doctor has a clear picture of the patient as a person. Equally, the patient must become aware of the doctor's identity. This mutual recognition of identity is the anchor of the doctor–patient relationship. It must be able to survive the many changes that time brings, such as ageing, disability or dementia. If doctor and patient can each say 'I know you – you are my doctor (or patient)', then trust and confidence can be maintained. The firmness of this relationship can help to offset the discontinuity of care that is inevitable should specialized, high-technology hospital care become necessary.

The multidisciplinary practice team is complementary to the recognition of identity between doctor and patient. Patients get to know the other doctors, nurses and lay staff, who all may come and go, but the practice continues as an entity. Can the practice sustain this notion of a corporate identity – of a friendly organization where people's dignity is respected, and there will be someone who is familiar and willing to help? Such continuity of corporate identity can only be achieved by longer-term planning and management than is usual in UK general practice. If the organization has a clear and empathic identity, then continuity of care may become a reality.

In an inner city with a high turnover of population, continuity would be more difficult to achieve. In some practices, over 25 per cent of patients change every year. In these circumstances the GP would be tempted to see the kaleidoscope of restless patients as a series of technical encounters, rather than as individuals, each living in their unique biographical time. Frankenberg (1988) summed up the different viewpoints of patient and doctor in a sentence: 'A woman is having a child – to the doctor she is a pregnant woman'. To the mother it is the start of a major long-term and unfolding story: to the doctor a nine-month responsibility – or sometimes just another 'case' of pregnancy.

The doctor's time apart from patients

Different settings, roles and domains
Demands on the general practitioner's time, and the patient's too, may come from a number of directions. So let us focus on the variety of settings in which GPs and patients operate, and the pressures to which they are subjected in various domains. Take the doctor first. He or she has the consultation as a major activity, coupled with home visits and practice administration. There are other professional activities, such as learning and teaching, outside jobs and medical politics. In the United Kingdom the time spent in the practice is not (in the main) directly linked to money, whereas outside jobs and teaching can generate revenue. They may generate conflict by giving GPs a financial incentive to spend time outside the practice at the expense of the everyday care of patients, but the variety may also enrich their lives and make them better doctors.

All the different work activities are in competition for time, and in contrast to the positive incentive of money, there is the negative incentive of avoiding the more stressful ways of spending time. The consultation stands out as an exacting activity (Porter et al., 1985). Home visiting is even more of a strain, as it is time-consuming, takes place on the patient's rather than the doctor's territory, is more likely to be an emergency and, in towns at least, there is the burden of urban traffic. No wonder that fewer home visits are now being done (Fry, 1983), and when list sizes become smaller, little of the time so freed is used to prolong the length of the consultation. Yet this may be a short-sighted policy, when an investment of time in greater rapport and more knowledge of the patient's problems and circumstances, might pay off in better care for the patient and less strain for the doctor.

The patient's life is similarly divided into domains competing for time, so a balance has somehow to be drawn between maximum time autonomy for both patient and doctor, and accountability for time as a scarce resource in a publicly funded service. This dilemma will be considered later. Meanwhile let us look at the different settings which concern doctors and patients and which compete for time. General practitioners, with unique perceptions of their own time and ways of organizing self time are surrounded by a number of areas of concern that operate in different time frames and compete for time, such as work and professional activity, the family, leisure, and the neighbour-hood. Patients are similarly placed but with their own unique per-ceptions of time and areas of concern, which may be very different to those of their doctor.

In the consultation, it can be assumed that the patient comes with something perceived as a 'health' problem, and likewise the doctor expects initially to be presented with a health problem. The doctor will need to be aware of factors in the patient's environment that determine health and illness, and which also compete for the patient's time and colour their perceptions of time. Each of the patient's domains may operate in different time frames and at very different rates to those of the doctor.

Time empathy

In the consultation, the doctor needs to understand what an illness means to the patient, and as a part of this process to appreciate what time means for the patient. Seeing things from the patient's viewpoint – 'getting in the patient's shoes' – must include the dimension of time. In the consultation this process of projection in order to gain under-standing is called empathy. In relation to seeing time as the patient sees it, the term 'time empathy' would seem to be appropriate.

This deeper understanding of the time problems experienced by patients could stem from GPs' deeper understanding of their own time problems, just as doctors who have had a particular illness can see better what the illness means to the patient. Understanding their own time problems in order to transfer this knowledge to the patient is only a first step, because the doctor's perceptions of time may be very different from the patient's. The GP may be brisk and efficient and a good 'time manager': the patient facing disability or death may see time quite differently. So the doctor will have to bridge this second gap by developing a deeper understanding of the patient's specific time problems as they affect health and illness. A close analogy is the effort needed by a normally affluent GP to understand what it is like to be poor and at a social disadvantage, or by a doctor from one culture making efforts to 'get inside' the beliefs and expectations of other cultures.

This poses the practical problem of helping the doctor to become aware of a patient's unique time perceptions, and the question as to whether any shortfall in understanding could be remedied by training. We now have to look at the various ways that time can be viewed in the context of general practice.

Kinds of time in general practice

Ways of looking at time
Most graphic models of human interactions and organizations are, perforce, spatial and static. Even time has to be represented spatially. Hence time is a neglected dimension. Hägerstrand (1985) in his pioneer work on time geography has gone a long way towards filling this gap, and his models link time to two-dimensional space. However, determinants of health and the workings of health care are multi-dimensional, and operate on several time scales both linear and cyclical (Young, 1988). The interactions of space and time are not considered in detail in this chapter as they have been well described in the context of general practice by Armstrong (1985).

Perhaps general practitioners could look to other disciplines such as sociology, social anthropology, time geography and economics for an understanding of time that would be relevant to sick people interacting with the health care team and with society.

People coin terms for the things that matter to them. Inuit are said to have a number of different words describing different kinds of ice, that are seen as distinct entities relevant to survival. So with time, many categories of time and metaphors for illuminating it have been described in literature and by philosophers and scientists, some of which may be useful to consider in the context of general practice.

Time as a commodity
This concept of time appeals to the general practitioner as an entrepreneur or 'tradesman', as opposed to 'priest' (Abel-Smith, 1976).

Time can be saved, spent, wasted, bought or invested or exchanged for money. It cannot be banked or recycled. Time is not money, but the relationship is closer in a 'fee-for-service' system of payment as opposed to salary or capitation. So the patient who pays will expect to have a greater call on the doctor's time, and so have a shorter wait. Buying better or more immediate health care is using the currency of money to exchange for the commodity of time. Countries which have encouraged a free service in monetary terms, may find it replaced by a service where time is the scarce commodity, and this can be manipulated for or against the patient's interests, just like money.

Economists talk about marginal cost, opportunity cost, cost efficiency and cost effectiveness. Substituting time for cost produces some useful categories. Marginal time indicates that extra work does not take so long as getting started, so that extra patients might be better accommodated in a flexible session, rather than running an additional session. Opportunity time refers to what could be done with time saved from other activities. Would it be spent wisely or wasted? When time management was discussed with GPs, they were asked what they would do with the time saved by efficiency, and most of them chose more time at home or at leisure. Very rarely did they choose to invest more time in the practice in order to lengthen the consultation time, lessen waiting or plan for the future.

'Not wasting time' has an authoritarian or puritan flavour which is linked to the ownership of time, and time efficiency. Whereas 'saving time' equates with Victorian ideas of goodness, 'borrowing time' may suggest short-term expedients to postpone the inevitable. However, to some extent, wasting time may be a form of relaxation and a way of lessening strain.

'Time efficiency' is the world of time management and the pocket organizer, of time-and-motion study and the tyranny of the stopwatch. Such methods imply a power gradient between managers and the managed, where managers' time is of greater value, so delegation 'pays off'. Time can be bought by employing extra staff and this alters the nature of the work both in terms of time spent and the intensity of work.

'Time effectiveness' relates time to the objectives of any activity and encourages a clear sense of the importance, urgency and priority of various tasks in order to achieve the aims of individuals or organizations. General practitioners are encouraged to improve their time effectiveness (RCGP, 1985), but it is not always clear whether this relates to their own aims or those of patients, which, as we have seen, are not necessarily congruent (Pritchard, 1981). GPs find courses on practice management more attractive when they focus on time and its problems. A recent distance-learning project on management for GPs and practice teams is entitled 'If only I had the time' (RCGP, 1989). However much we may believe that by sorting out objectives, priorities and procedures, time will look after itself, time is a powerful motivating factor for change which cannot be ignored if it encourages GPs to look critically at the way they work, and to relate time to their own and their patients' aims and values.

Social time

Jaques (1982) produced an impressive formulation of social time in contrast to clock/calendar time, using a two-dimensional model. On one scale is the inexorably ticking clock or moving calendar. These link past with present and future in a physical sense, and allow modern life to function, with its coordination and timing of events. But this is not the way we think nor act if we can avoid it. The other dimension of social or 'intention time' is directed towards one's goals and aspirations, and is marked more as a succession of events, with time passing quickly or slowly according to the intensity of the activity or experience. Past events are remembered primarily in social time, and only linked to calendar time when there is a particular reason for doing so.

'Self time' or 'personal time' includes one's own pacemaker, for the heart as well as for other biorhythms, and it sets the pace of one's life. It is complex and unique – difficult enough to understand in oneself, but even more so for doctor and patient to understand each other's self time. If there can be some harmonizing of the doctor's and patient's self time, one might postulate that time empathy will be easier to achieve. But a serious disharmony might make empathy more difficult to establish, unless doctors could learn to be less conscious of their own pace of life in order to identify more closely with the patients'. So the 'doctor in a hurry' could adjust deliberately to the patient's pace – the doctor could be 'walking in step'.

'Time out' is when people escape from the trap of conflict with time in order to relax and enjoy themselves. Time then has a different quality of refreshment – of relieving rather than generating strain. Time out for thinking, for creative activity and for laughing also has a different quality to working time. Unless given a high priority, it tends to be crowded out. Yet 'thinking time' is essential to ensure that values, goals and priorities are clearly perceived and ordered. Creative activity can give a new purpose and refreshment to life and so make the more humdrum daily use of time more tolerable.

But sickness, unemployment, terminal illness and death may be seen as time out of a different kind, when other rules apply. People have to adapt to harsh temporal reality, but are GPs aware of the lethal consequences of sick and workless roles so that they may give appropriate help? Doctors may find it hard to appreciate that most life is led in disregard of mortality. Though we all have to die, any moment seems open-ended. But to the sick patient, whose life may be or is actually threatened, time becomes a closed and finite dimension. In terminal illness, time is running out, so in a sense is more precious, but not if it is purposeless or spent in pain. Doctors may be able to help to make sick and workless time more purposeful and terminal time more serene.

Social or intention time as noted before, progresses at a variable rate according to the value placed on the event. Time flies when we are busy or happy, and drags when we are sad of idle, or the task is pointless. When time flies happily we are unconscious of it, but time may also disappear when we are desperately short of it and working under pressure. This consciousness of 'time intensity', whether it flies or drags, is an example of a disharmony with clock time that distorts our perception of its passing.

Sometimes, at moments of intense experience, time has a different quality which imprints itself firmly on our memory, as when some people remember exactly what they were doing when some important or historic event occurred. In the consultation, doctors and patients sometimes experience a vivid moment of insight – the 'flash' (Balint, 1973) – that gives a fresh view of the nature of the problem, and produces an emotional rapport as well.

Time structures
'Biographical time' or life's path gives both a linear and cyclical account of an individual's passage from birth, through school, work or child rearing and retirement to death. When two individuals are closely linked like husband and wife or twins, they may assume a joint biography, because the narrative does not end when one of them dies, but when the survivor dies. In the period of bereavement, time will have lost much of its structure and meaning. Time will have been embedded mutually in joint events, which become insupportable alone. Family records in general practice could enhance the concept of shared biographical time.

Biographical time is of particular importance in general practice, where medical history is crucial to diagnosis, and the interrelationships of events must be fixed with precision. Some of this biography is in the patient's medical record, but most of the communication between doctor and patient is oral, and little of this is recorded. The main repository of the patient's medical biography will be the memory of the personal doctor. This is another compelling reason for personal doctoring as a way of sharing in each other's biographical time. Otherwise people will be reluctant to share their secrets, and general practice could become more restricted to the technical domain, rather than serve a wider range of patients' needs.

Just as the daily routine is embedded in weekly, monthly, seasonal and annual routines so are temporal events embedded in each other. A consultation is embedded in the session and in the day. The patient sees the doctor in the middle of several other time-dependent activities, like working, shopping, catching the bus home, or fetching children from school. If they intrude on each other, frustration occurs leading to tension. The allocation of time between different roles and domains that interrelate is an example of 'embedded time' of considerable complexity.

'Interaction time' describes the time that doctor and patient are available to interact, and this may only average about 25 minutes a year. But how they interact also has a temporal dimension, in giving the other time to speak. Communication has been shown to work best when the patient does most of the talking initially, and the doctor taking over later in the consultation (Ley, 1983).

'Team time' is a useful reminder that teamwork requires a disciplined approach to punctuality, a shared sense of urgency, and time empathy focused on the organization as well as on individuals. Experience has shown that the different senses of urgency which are customary in different professions are a potent source of conflict (Huntington, 1981).

Habits and routines

Young (1988) in *The Metronomic Society* describes habits as 'the flywheel of society'. This metaphor suggests that we can coast along with the flywheel providing the energy, so that we do not have to think out repeated actions each time. Without it, Young argues, life would be very exhausting. Experienced general practitioners can take short cuts and rely on habits when – say – prescribing for common diseases. Yet habits can be a serious pitfall for the unwary. Diseases may have similar patterns, but patients tend to be unique in their nature and their problems. To ignore this could lead to 'slot machine' medicine, where stereotyped groups of symptoms might evoke an automatic response. Even computerized decision support systems do not fall into this trap (Fox et al., 1990). They have complex logical pathways and may consider 50 or more hypotheses in a relatively straightforward case. Always, the decision is left to the doctor not the machine.

Because each consultation is unique, great concentration is needed by both doctor and patient and it is tiring for both. To rely on the flywheel of habit as a source of energy would be risky. Habitual responses may, however, be appropriate in the early stages of a consultation, when rapport is being established. When doctor and patient know each other well, they can dive straight in to where they were last time, without first having to test the water. Given a knowledge of each other's habits and mutual trust, much time can be saved.

The clock and calendar have long been symbols of power – of the need of religions or employers to control the time of others, as well as giving humans more control over their environment in husbandry and navigation. Bureaucratic time is the imposed structure of an organized society, and finds expression in timetables, career structures and routines. Though necessary to a degree, it is a ready vehicle for the exercise of power. In a bureaucratic health service the likely result is longer waiting time for patients and less opportunity for choice.

General practitioners are able to enhance their already substantial power by manipulating time. Appointment systems that were designed to help patients may have had a contrary effect in confirming that the doctor is busy and that patients will have to wait for an appointment unless it is urgent, as judged by someone other than the patient. This devalues and disempowers the patient. Only a few doctors will deny that they are busy, and this may be viewed with suspicion by their peers. This dilemma cannot easily be resolved since conscientious doctors need to occupy their time, but not appear too busy. The power gradient is difficult to level because it is hard to resist power when it is offered on a plate by polite patients telling doctors how busy they are. For doctors and staff just to recognize that time is an expression of power would be a step forward.

The tacit medical ownership of the time spent interacting with patients is strongest in a hospital setting and weakest when visiting the patient's home, with the surgery appointment somewhere in between. With home visiting now much less frequent, appointment systems becoming the norm, hospital referral (in general) on the increase, and fewer people dying in their homes, patients can expect to suffer an increasing loss of power and capacity to control their own time. This subtle spatial and temporal shift in their place of care works against the apparent consensus that patients should have more opportunity for self-reliance and management of their own health and illness.

The central paradox is that doctors who become convinced that they are busy people without enough time, automatically forfeit their time autonomy and the freedom that goes with it. By accepting the power of control over other people's time, they may lose control of their own self time – itself a source of power.

'Waiting time' has many causes, and is a good measure of the powerlessness of the patient. It is an indicator of the balance of power in an organization, and in general practice there should be no excuse for patients having to wait for more than two days to see a doctor, and a same-day service should be available on the patient's request, not in the gift of the receptionist.

Waiting is a learned response against a natural impatience and need to get things done to suit oneself, so it represents a conflict between self time and other time. For example in conversation each must wait for the other to speak in order to communicate, but waiting is built in to the structure of our society, and is an expression of power. The powerless wait for the powerful. When there is no need to wait, but people are made to 'cool their heels', this becomes a 'ritual degradation' (Weigert, 1981). Waiting for appointments, in clinics and for admission to hospital, is increasingly becoming the norm in the National Health Service. When people pay for private health care in the United Kingdom, they are mainly paying to avoid the uncertainty of waiting.

If doctors are really aiming to treat patients as equals, then there must be a balanced negotiation of time as of other expressions of power. This implies a participative approach to sharing power that is not popular with professions, but is slowly gaining ground. Participation evokes a warm response in patients (Pritchard, 1981), so it could be argued that patients would be more cooperative if they had not been kept waiting.

A health care system with no waiting whatever would be too difficult to design. But patients will often accept waiting if they know how long it is likely to be and an explanation is given for the reason for the delay. Equally, waiting times can be manipulated to implement policies and priorities, but not without negotiation with the patient whose body and time it is.

A summary of kinds of time

Are all these kinds of time just literary abstractions, or do they have meaning, and represent discernible categories and distinctions? Alas, the varieties are not clear-cut, and overlap too much for a coherent classification. However certain classes and dimensions of time do emerge, and some sort of spectrum or power-shift diagram might be constructed, but it could not fit in all the kinds of time. Social or intention time as opposed to clock or calendar time can be grasped as a two-dimensional matrix – with perhaps a third dimension of 'time as information' (Michon, 1985). Some kinds of time, such as self time, time out and time empathy, can be linked to autonomy and freedom; others are part of social control, for example clock time, bureaucratic and waiting time and time as power. Time structures include time as a commodity, interaction time, embedded time and biographical time. They can be seen as linking the other dimensions of autonomy or control.

Time is not so easy to see, feel and measure as space, so metaphors are used. In a sense, all the ways of looking at time are metaphors. Doctors and patients may use quite different metaphors for self time. A doctor may see him- or herself as a knight in shining armour riding to bring succour to a maiden in distress, or crossing the boundaries of space and time like Superman. Sick patients may view themselves as floating passively on a sluggish stream towards oblivion.

The difficulty is to balance the two extremes of autonomy and control in each domain at each moment. Who should control the doctor's time? Should it be mainly self-controlled, controlled by patients or by bureaucrats? In the United Kingdom, doctors have a large measure of control of their own time, though patient-demand moderates some of this. Yet UK doctors, as stated earlier, spend least time with patients. In Canada and the United States where patients pay fees, they assume a measure of control, yet demand is satisfied more by the market than by legislation. In Nordic countries, especially Finland, there would seem to be more bureaucratic control of time, yet waiting times build up, and doctors and patients may be unhappy.

The general practitioner as an initiator of change?

The problems
Several problem areas for GPs have been described such as short consultations giving an episodic view of the trajectory of illness; the altered time perceptions in illness; the difficulty GPs have in understanding people's time frames even when they are well, let alone when time is distorted by illness. Some of these problems might be alleviated by organizational change, others would need changes in individual GP's knowledge, skills and attitudes.

Organizational change
Much can be achieved by conscious attempts by doctors and staff to produce a patient-oriented organization in which patients' time and convenience is given greater value, waiting time is reduced, and consultation time increased to a mutually acceptable level. In one practice (Harrison, 1987), patients were given the choice of how much time they would like booked for their next appointment, and their estimates proved very accurate. Certain features of general practice help the doctor to understand the time dimension of health and one of these is a long-term doctor–patient relationship. So the personal doctor system (Gray, 1979) is one key, and this is helped by stability of doctors' work and patients' domicile.

Some practices are beginning to look further ahead and record their aims and achievements in practice annual reports (Gray, 1985). Sharing the information in these reports with patients, and ensuring that time, both patients' and doctors', is not forgotten, will encourage the development of an empathic 'learning organization' (Coates and Evans, 1987), where patients' real concerns are not dismissed as trivia. This kind of organization will be able to adapt to change more readily in spite of turbulence in the environment.

Personal change

Of all the concepts mentioned in this paper, the deliberate attempt to understand time from the patient's viewpoint – described as 'time empathy' – might be usefully introduced into medical education in order to alert both doctors and patients to the necessity of bridging the perception gap. Learning to practise 'time empathy', though difficult, would be in line with current trends in training GPs to develop a more patient-centred consulting style. To this could be added a deeper understanding of time as another dimension of perception and experience – for both doctor and patient. GPs in training could be helped by learning a suitable repertoire for eliciting the patient's time problems, just as they have to learn a repertoire for taking a medical or psychiatric history. Making explicit the metaphors that both doctors and patients use to describe time might be a way of exploring and developing time empathy. But central to the understanding of patients' time and managing time effectively is self-knowledge and an appreciation of the complex workings of time both in individuals and in society.

Disciplines such as sociology, social anthropology and psychology have progressed much further along this path of inquiry than has general practice, so a transfer of learning might be fruitful. This chapter has tried to outline the sorts of knowledge and ideas that might help general practitioners to come to terms with their own time and tune in to their patients' time, and that of the primary health care team. But they should not bear this responsibility alone. Many of the decisions that doctors make require an understanding of issues of social policy that they do not possess, and a dialogue across the artificial boundaries of disciplines could only be of benefit to patients and doctors.

Notes

I should like to acknowledge with thanks the help I have been freely given in the preparation of this chapter by Barbara Adam, Edgar Borgenhammer, Ronald Frankenberg, Mayer Hillman, John Horder, Laurie McMahon, Wendy Pritchard, Ann Richardson, Tom Schuller and Wendy Stainton Rogers. June Huntington, David Pendleton and Michael Young have been fruitful sources of ideas for which I am grateful. Sue Flanders processed the text.

References

Abel-Smith, B. (1976) *Value for money in health services*. London: Heinemann. Chapter 5.

Arber, S. and Sawyer, L. (1979) 'Changes in the structure of general practice: the patient's viewpoint', evidence to the Royal Commission on the National Health Service. London: DHSS.

Armstrong, D. (1985) 'Space and time in British general practice', *Social Science and Medicine*, 20: 659–66.

Balint, E. (1973) 'The "flash" technique – its freedom and its discipline', E. Balint and J. Norell (eds), *Six minutes for the patient*. London: Tavistock.

Bradley, N.C.A. (1983) 'Time and the general practice consultation', in D.J. Pereira Gray (ed.), *Medical Annual 1983*. Bristol: Wright PSG. pp. 254–61.

Cartwright, A. (1967) *Patients and their doctors. A study of general practice*. London: Routledge and Kegan Paul.

Cartwright, A. and Anderson, R. (1981) *General practice revisited. A second study of patients and their doctors*. London: Tavistock.

Coates, R. and Evans, K. (1987) 'The learning organization', in B. Stocking (ed.), *In dreams begins responsibility*. London: King's Fund.

DHSS (1987) *Workload in general practice*. A report prepared for the Doctors' and Dentists' Review Body 1985/6. London: HMSO. pp. 254–61.

Donald, A.G. (1985) 'Oasis or beachhead', James Mackenzie lecture 1985, *Journal of the Royal College of General Practitioners*, 35: 581–61.

Fox, J., Glowinski, A., Gordon, C., Hajnal, S. and O'Neil, M. (1990) 'Logic engineering for knowledge engineering: design and implementation of the Oxford System of Medicine', *Artificial Intelligence in Medicine*, 2: 323–39.

Frankenberg, R. (1988) ' "Your time or mine?" ', An anthropological view of the tragic temporal contradictions of biomedical practice', in M. Young and T. Schuller (eds), *The Rhythms of Society*. London: Routledge.

Fry, J. (1983) *Present state and future needs in general practice*, 6th edn, Royal College of General Practitioners. Lancaster: MTP Press.

Gray, D.J. Pereira (1979) 'The key to personal care', *Journal of the Royal College of General Practitioners*, 29: 666–78.

Gray, D.J. Pereira (1985) 'Practice annual reports', in *The Medical Annual 1985*. Bristol: Wright PSG.

Hägerstrand, T. (1985) 'Time and culture', in G. Kirsch et al. (eds), *Time Preferences: an interdisciplinary and empirical approach*. Berlin: Wissenschaftszentrum.

Harrison, A.T. (1987) 'Appointment systems: feasibility study of a new approach', *British Medical Journal*, 294: 1465–6.

Hull, F.M. (1983) 'The GP's use of time: an international comparison', Update, 1 April 1983: 1243–53.

Huntington, J. (1981) 'Time orientations in the collaboration of social workers and general practitioners', *Social Science and Medicine*, 15A: 203.

Jaques, E. (1982) *The form of time*. London: Heinemann.

Jones, J.W. (ed.) (1981) *The burnout syndrome*. Illinois: London House Management Press.

Ley, P. (1983) 'Patients' understanding and recall in clinical communication' in D. Pendleton and J. Hasler (eds), *Doctor–Patient communication*. London: Academic Press. pp. 89–107.

Michon, J.A. (1985) 'The compleat time experience', in J.A. Michon and J.L. Jackson (eds), *Time, Mind and Behaviour*. Berlin: Springer Verlag. pp. 20–52.

Morrell, D.C., Evans, M.E., Morris, R.W. and Roland, M.O. (1986) 'The "five minute" consultation: effect of time constraint on clinical content and patient satisfaction', *British Medical Journal*, 292: 870–3.

Porter, A.M.D., Howie, J.G.R. and Levinson, A. (1985) 'Measurement of stress as it affects the work of the general practitioner', *Family Practice*, 2: 136–46.

Pritchard, P.M.M. (1981) *Manual of primary health care: its nature and organization*, 2nd edn. Oxford: Oxford University Press. pp. 17, 118.

Pritchard, P.M.M. (1986) 'Participation', in J. Fry and J. Hasler (eds), *Primary Health Care 2000*. Edinburgh: Churchill Livingstone. pp. 84–100.

RCGP (1985) *Quality in General Practice*. Policy Statement No 2. London: Royal College of General Practitioners. p. 8.

RCGP (1989) *'If only I had the time!' an introduction to better management in practice*. Royal College of General Practitioners and Centre for Medical Education, University of Dundee.

Social Research Unit, NOP Market Research Ltd (1982) Health poll. The public's use of and attitudes towards GPs. London: NOP Market Research Ltd.

Weigert, A.J. (1981) *Sociology of everyday life*. London: Longman.

Wilkin, D., Hodgkin, P. and Metcalfe, D. (1986) 'Factors affecting workload: is received wisdom true?' in D.J. Gray Pereira (ed.), *The Medical Annual 1986*. Bristol: Wright PSG. pp. 185–96.

Young, M. (1988) *The Metronomic Society: natural rhythms and human timetables*. London: Thames and Hudson.

6
Time and the Hospital Consultant

Ken Starkey

The commodification of time is a dominant feature of capitalist society in which economic order depends upon the control of time. This commodification is encapsulated in the dictum 'time is money'. Thinking of time as a commodity and as a scarce resource has led to the quantification of time, made possible by the clock which is perhaps the key machine of industrial society. Mumford (1973) emphasizes this point when he stresses that the primary characteristic of modern machine civilization is its aspiration to temporal regularity, made possible by the clock. Weber (1976) sees the rationalization of time as a fundamental characteristic of the Spirit of Capitalism. Time is the primary scarce resource. A key task of managerial work is to make sure that time is not wasted. Time thus becomes an important area of potential conflict at work (Thompson, 1967; Starkey, 1986). Time is an important element of the employment contract and a key area of negotiation between employer and employee in the definition of work roles. Time is always too short for management and too long for labour. Management tries to control time in order to prolong it while labour tries to control time in order to shorten it (Gurvitch, 1963: 44). Management looks to maximize the productive use of time. Historically this maximization was done by extending the length of the working day. When this became impossible and the working day started to reduce in length management turned to the intensification of time use and getting the most out of the time that was available through more sophisticated forms of managerial monitoring and control.

In this chapter we examine the nature of thinking about time in medical work as exemplified in contrasting views of what is the appropriate form of contract to govern the work of medical professionals. Time has been a key issue in hospital consultants' attempts to define the nature of their commitments to the National Health Service. It has also been a key element in employers' attempts to define what they see as the correct nature of this commitment. Differing perceptions of the nature of temporal commitment formed the substance of the contract dispute between consultants and the Department of Health and Social Security that persisted throughout most of the 1970s. It is an assertion of this chapter that the issues raised in this dispute have never been satisfactorily resolved. The nature of consultants' temporal commitment remains, at best, imprecise. Imprecision lies at the very heart of the medical contract.

Time, work and contract

In his classic study of the nature of the employment contract Fox (1974) examines the relationship between contract, power relations and trust relations between employer and employee. Fox distinguishes between two forms of exchange relationship – social and economic – and describes a trend towards economic relationships at work. Economic exchange, he argues, engenders low trust relations. It depends on the formalization of accountability governed by a closed contract which functions as a managerial control device. It leaves low discretion to the employee in the performance of work. Its enforcement depends on close supervision and bureaucratic rules designed to monitor performance. The work contract based on economic exchange is job-specific. It represents the power of management to impose its work designs. The worker 'supplies explicitly specified services' (ibid.: 178). The effect of this explicitness is to curtail 'diffuse obligations'. The worker reacts to the low trust placed in him or her by refusing to give more than the contract stipulates. The explicit contract tends towards the maximum definition of what is expected of the employee.

A more open form of contract based on high trust relations between employer and employee leaves contractual obligations on the employee's part very open and the nature of the trust relation is such that the employee is prepared to give more as his or her side of the employment bargain. This is the basis of Fox's opposite to economic exchange – social exchange. Social exchange depends on personal obligation not impersonal bureaucratic rules and on employee discretion in an unsupervised work situation. Reciprocity is expected but is not precisely defined as it is in economic exchange. The occupant of the high-discretion role participates in a community based on moral obligation not calculative expediency and pure market exchange (ibid.: 83, 289).

Fox views contract and its evolutionary tendency towards principles of economic exchange as a managerial control device aimed at 'the redefining of roles in terms of minimum discretion' (ibid.: 62). A key element of the employment contract relates to time. This concerns that portion of the contract that defines the 'geometry' of working time (Grossin, 1969) – the duration of working time and the different segments that constitute this duration. Management is character-

istically concerned with the management of time and with the control
of how employers use their time. It is a managerial assumption of
economic exchange that employees, unless tightly controlled in the
way they use their time, will tend to 'free-load'. Conversely occupational groups typically attempt to structure their time use in their
own best interests (Gurvitch, 1963). Just as management can attempt
to extract greater effort by more precise temporal specification of
duties as in scientific management reference to contract by occupational groups can be used as a strategy by employees for controlling
the wage-effort bargain (Baldamus, 1961). 'Work-to-rules' are the
classic mode of this employee strategy. The rules specify a degree of
time commitment and this precision of usage. Employees refuse
activity that is not so defined.

Professionals and time

Fox sees low-trust relations predominating in rank and file production
work and contrasts this with professional work. The worker in the
former 'has little sense of being an expert; of commitment to a calling;
of autonomy on the job; or of obligation to produce high quality work;
in other words, of being a professional' (Fox, 1974: 29). The specification of duties excludes choice which the professional retains.
Professional obligations are diffuse:

> The ideology of professionalism defines the work to be so extraordinarily
> complex and non-routine that the profession must be allowed to exercise its
> own independent judgement over how the work is organized.... While
> members of most occupations seek to be free to control the level and
> direction of their work efforts, it is distinct to professionalism to assert that
> such freedom is a necessary condition for the proper performance of work.
> (Freidson, 1970: 153–4.

When professionals are involved the management of time becomes
particularly problematic as professionals rarely recognize the managerial prerogative as legitimate in the definition of the best way of
allocating their time. Professionals are not subject to the same level of
temporal constraint that weighs on other less privileged occupational
groups. In particular they are not subject to the same degree of time
discipline, symbolized by the need to conform to the dictates of clock
time. Professionals are free to organize themselves according to a
'calendar of tasks' rather than a 'formal calendar of hours of work'
(Lamour and Chalendar, 1974: 108).

An alternative view of professional time suggests that their privilege
has been exaggerated and that once professionals enter work in large
bureaucratic organizations they inevitably become subject to the
temporal rules of these organizations. The routinization of work in this

way is seen as an inevitable tendency of modern forms of work. Professional status gives way to employee status. Employee status implies conformity to the organizational rules and routines of which temporal routines are particularly important in the pursuit of economic efficiency. Professionals run the risk of losing a large degree of their independent status. Management begins to whittle away at their privileges. Accountability and control increase. In large organizations it is technocrats not professionals who set the rules (Heydebrand, 1983). Professional and managerial/organizational logics collide head-on. Zerubavel, one of the most perceptive writers on time in modern society, argues that this is a major social trend: 'One of the most significant aspects of the rationalization of social life in modern Western civilization is the increasing bureaucratization of professional commitments, which is clearly manifested through the rigidification of their temporal boundaries' (Zerubavel, 1981: 159).

The hospital consultants' contract dispute

In professional work the time aspect of contract has not until recently been precisely defined. Contracts have been open-ended. This lack of definition has led to increasing contractual problems for hospital consultants and their employers. A generalized dissatisfaction among hospital consultants with the way their time is managed came to a head in the contract dispute of the 1970s between consultants and their ultimate paymaster, the government, represented by the Department of Health and Social Security (DHSS). The nature of the contract, it was argued by the profession, created major time problems – primarily too long working hours and too diffuse temporal commitments. The profession argued for a more closely defined contract to replace what they saw as a contract that was too open-ended in terms of time-commitment.

> This demand arose partly through the feeling among maximum part-timers that they were being exploited by being required to provide a service as great as whole-timers at a substantially lower salary, but also from whole-timers who found the demands made upon them were increasing steadily. (*British Medical Journal*, 16 June 1979: 1653)

The demand led to a confrontation between consultants and the government that lasted from 1974 to 1979, the issues raised in which are still, as we move into the 1990s and a period of great change in the way the National Health Service is managed with a move towards market forms of management, unresolved.

Central to the dispute of the 1970s were differing definitions of the relevant time commitments consultants should bring to their work and central to these definitions was the concept of clinical responsibility and arguments as to whether this should be of an open or closed form, that is, all-embracing or limited to set, contracted times. Other grades of doctor were also dissatisfied with time aspects of their work. While the consultant dispute continued, junior hospital doctors went as far as taking strike action over hours of work which were, they argued, 'reminiscent of the nineteenth century' (Gordon and Iliffe, 1977: 6). Again, this particular issue remains unresolved at the beginning of the 1990s with junior doctors still militating for reductions in their working hours during their time in the training grades. Consultants, too, were saying that the existing open-ended contract with no specified time parameters, only an open commitment to total responsibility for the patients under their care, was no longer appropriate to medical work and late-twentieth-century working conditions of service.

Not all consultants agreed with this view. Arguments over the issue raged, not only between the consultants as a body and their paymaster (the DHSS), but between consultants themselves. A minority felt that attitudes towards time which they regarded as reminiscent of trade unions were not appropriate to a profession whose necessary level of commitment could not be fitted into the standard hours of an industrial-type contract. Interestingly, academic clinicians employed in universities spoke particularly strongly against a more closed form of contract. The profession's official representatives, however, were not averse to flexing their 'industrial muscle' as 'the only way if doctors are to keep afloat in today's inflationary society' (Gordon and Iliffe, 1977: 41). Issues of working time were inextricably linked to issues of pay bargaining. A key goal for the profession's pay negotiators was a contract that was more work-sensitive in its effects on pay than the existing open contract, a contract which, while not over-defined, was precise enough in its definition of minimal time commitments to permit a large increase in pay which would enable the profession to regain the differentials that it had lost in previous pay-bargaining rounds. The DHSS wanted a contract that was closed on its terms, specifying a Monday to Friday 9.00 am to 5.00 pm week of ten four-hour sessions rather than notional sessions, the Notional Half Days (NHDs) specified in consultants' contracts (*British Medical Journal*, 4 January 1975: 45). The DHSS felt that some consultants, particularly the part-timers, were not fulfilling their obligations to the NHS and the new contract was designed to tighten controls.

A key point in both consultant and junior doctors' disputes was the nature of professional commitment. Resistance to the junior doctors' action in pursuit of a new contractual status relative to time on the job was couched in terms of such demands being 'unprofessional'. Gordon and Iliffe (1977) argue that the hidden agenda here was not professionalism per se but the more pragmatic recognition that the consequences of a dilution of the concept of professionalism would be that junior medical staff would no longer provide unpaid labour solely on the basis of commitment considered appropriate to the professional. The issue of consultants' time was more complex ideologically as consultants themselves clung to the notion of professionalism in their resistance to the government version of a closed contract, arguing that the nature of professional work was incompatible with fixed hours, while at the same time holding the notion of professionalism in abeyance when it came to a close definition of the nature of their responsibilities in temporal terms.

Monitoring the situation and trying to translate negotiation into pay recommendations was the Review Body on Doctors' and Dentists' Remuneration (the DDRB) which argued that professionalism and salaries related directly to length of working hours were incompatible: 'It is inappropriate to relate professional salaries to length of working hours' (DDRB, 1977: para. 2.3). The DDRB argued that a set salary was the appropriate form of reumuneration for professional work and that extra item-of-service payments and overtime-type payments were totally inappropriate. The profession adopted a dual strategy, walking a fine line between assertions of professional autonomy and the specification of 'out of hours' payments of the kind found in industry. Starting from the assertion that their earnings had seen a marked decline relative to other occupational groups they proceeded to link this with the argument that a large part of their work for the NHS was, in fact, voluntary and unpaid because it was conducted at times over and above their contracted hours. This they saw as an abuse of their good faith and used as the basis of their militating for a more closely defined workload sensitive contract. As a form of action to support their case they proposed a 'work to contract'.

The new contract sought by the profession constituted a mix of sessional, emergency recall and on-call payments. It was to function in terms not of a timetable 'with its spectre of clocking on and off' (DDRB, 1978: para. 33) but according to a 'work schedule' over which the profession was to be the final arbiter. It differed from the old, open-ended contract in the extent to which aspects of the work previously covered by salary were to be separately contracted and paid for. It met the profession's three major objectives. First, it limited the open-ended commitment of the old contract in defining what time commitment was covered and thus specifying when extra payments for extra duties were applicable, though the profession was explicit in stating that it did not regard 'the definition of individual contracts as synonymous with their closure' (*British Medical Journal*, 22 February 1975: 471). The consultant was still free to define when and what extra time was needed. Second, the contract guaranteed adequate remuneration for

NHS work by providing payment for work performed beyond contractual commitments. And, third, it allowed consultants to do as they wished outside of their contracted hours. This time was now formally defined as 'free time'. The profession did not see this more precise definition of contractual responsibility as the abnegation or, indeed, any limitation of clinical responsibility or concern. The Royal Commission on the NHS, though, expressed grave concern that this new form of contract constituted a step towards regarding work as an optional activity, as 'a favour to the patient rather than being part of the normal business of providing care' (Royal Commission, 1979, para. 14: 72). The new contract could be seen as subversive of the traditional consultant role of providing total care regardless of time. The Royal Commission also considered the new contract to be unprofessional. For the profession's negotiators it constituted, not a subversion, but, rather, an 'identification' of a standard working week against which extra time commitments could be measured and remunerated. It was not, they argued, a limitation of professional concern. The quality, and indeed, the quantity of care was not to be diluted. It was merely to be adequately remunerated.

Some members of the profession suggested that the new contract might constitute, in the long run, a pyrrhic victory, facilitating a subsequent imposition of the dreaded closed contract. The profession would have to claim and justify overtime payments which would thus be open to administrative scrutiny. This could be construed as the first step towards the quantification of work and the specification of time norms for standard forms of activity which would eventually lead to the erosion of the professional freedom to allocate time to clinical, teaching, research and managerial activities as the individual consultant saw fit without interference from the employing authority. The door might thus be opened to the DHSS setting norms for the number of patients to be seen and treated per session and the regulation of treatment and discharge schedules (*British Medical Journal*, 1 January 1977: 53). The contract dispute in fact ended when the new contract was rejected by the profession at the eleventh hour on the grounds of its pricing. It was realized by the profession that emergency recall fees were not being budgeted for separately and would have to come out of the global sum allocated for all elements of the wage settlement for the year. The settlement would, therefore, tend to penalize those with few recall commitments while those with potentially heavy such commitments, for example surgeons, stood to gain at the expense of their colleagues. The only change to the contract actually implemented was to permit maximum whole-time consultants to undertake private work.

Developments in the 1980s

For Fox the benefits of advance towards explicit contract are asymmetrical. He sees the development of explicit contractual relations as evidence of a shift in power to employers. In professional work this would constitute a shift in the frontier of control away from professional autonomy and an example of deprofessionalization. Some social theorists see deprofessionalization as the trend of the future and predict that professionals' control of their work will be challenged on its 'three basic dimensions of special knowledge, service and autonomy' (Haug, 1973: 199). The medical profession, for example, has traditionally enjoyed a large advantage in defining the agendas concerning health care. The problems of the NHS have tended to be defined from its point of view in terms of shortage of resources:

> The medical profession therefore escape all blame for the shortcomings of the service and virtually remove from the agenda all examination of how existing resources are used or misused. Governments, the Treasury, the DHSS become the villains to be blamed. The central problem of clinical freedom and resources remains safely off the agenda. (Wilding, 1982: 30)

The profession justifies demands for extra resources on the grounds of the discrepancy between what medicine can do and what it is allowed to do by the resources it is allocated by the state.

Medical hegemony is increasingly under attack. Ongoing reorganisation of the NHS, represented by the Griffiths Report (NHS Management Inquiry, 1983) and the 1989 White Paper *Working For Patients*, represents attempts to reconceptualize the ground rules of medical care, primarily by substituting 'explicit public accounting' for the profession's 'implicit responsibility' for providing an efficient service (Wilding, 1982: 147–8). The starting point for the Griffiths Report is the weakness of the NHS caused by the lack of a clearly defined management function covering planning and performance appraisal. Griffiths 'suggests that most of the weaknesses in NHS management – imprecise objectives, little measurement of health output, infrequent evaluation of performance against agreed clinical, social and economic criteria – flow from this general organisational defect' (House of Commons Social Services Committee, 1984: 179). General managers are recommended to rectify the weakness by providing the managerial control that the NHS has historically lacked. The Report also stresses the need for acceptance by clinicians that the allocation of resources is related 'to priority needs in the population and to some acceptable level of cost and effectiveness' (NHS Management Inquiry, 1983: 130). The profession is urged to come to terms with the limits on clinical autonomy that are implicit in finite resources: 'The most critical issue of all is the sense among clinicians that there is pressure on resources, that they cannot expect any radical change for the better, and that as a consequence of this realisation they develop cooperative rather than competitive modes of behaviour' (NHS Management Inquiry, 1983: 130) in their negotiations about resource allocation.

The 1989 White Paper argues for the introduction of market forces into the National Health Service. It defines the duty of the health authorities as one of contracting for the best possible services and the best value for money from its own hospitals, from other authorities, from the newly created self-governing hospitals or from the private sector. The general practitioner is given the key role of acting as the patient's representative, as his or her 'agent', in seeking out the best quality and the quickest treatment. It is the hospital consultant who is the greatest consumer of health resources. The general practitioner's expanded role can be construed as an attempt to limit the power of the consultants. The 1989 reorganization of health services differed fundamentally from earlier reorganizations in the Department of Health's studied non-consultation with the medical profession over the kinds of changes to be introduced (Klein, 1990).

In the 1980s the problem of contract was still to the forefront of the evolving – some would say, including perhaps a majority of clinicians, increasingly vexed – relationship between clinicians and management. With the Short Report and the avowed intention to reduce the number of doctors in junior medical grades, consultants have expressed concern that they will inevitably be faced with extra work as numbers in their teams are reduced. There have also been problems in some health authorities where management has insisted that some elements of consultants' work, in particular on-call commitments, cannot be considered as time worked and thus used to reduce commitments to work other clinical sessions. Some authorities have also demanded that consultants complete work schedules to demonstrate the nature of their working patterns. The profession has responded by stipulating, on its side, what it considers a 'standard week'. Professional associations have advised their members accordingly and the Faculty of Anaesthetists and the Royal College of Obstetricians and Gynaecologists have gone as far as setting out in writing norms for average working patterns in terms of such measures as operating sessions and patients per clinic. The House of Commons Public Accounts Committee has recently argued that more control needs to be exercised over consultant neglect of NHS commitments by introducing more precise job definitions (*British Medical Journal*, 4 August 1990: 255). The consultant contract is currently being renegotiated 'to show who does what, where and when' (*British Medical Journal*, 3 February 1990: 290).

Conclusion

Proponents of a thesis of increasing professionalization of work argue that the future world of work will be characterized by a transition from the principle of managerial authority to professional authority, operating through self-discipline and the internalization of the norms of professional ideology rather than the external imposition of control and its monitoring by management (Halmos, 1973). Proponents of a deprofessionalization thesis argue that, on the contrary, professional autonomy is a dwindling phenomenon. Professionals are coming increasingly 'under the aegis of the state' (Esland, 1980: 229–30) which is the ultimate paymaster both for salaries and for the technology that makes their work possible. According to the deprofessionalization thesis a deterioration in the professional condition is inevitable given cuts in state expenditure and other symptoms of the fiscal crisis of the state (O'Connor, 1972). Professional rationales for the use of resources are weak, anyway, when the supply of those resources depends on external provision (Elliott, 1975). The rationing of services is the growing logic governing the management of state provision. The context is growing resource constraint and attacks on slack exemplified by the Audit Commission's report on further education.

The Audit Commission's Report (1985) on further education can be seen as a prime example of the direction in which the state would like to move in the definition of appropriate ways of organizing and controlling professional time. Contracts in further education were re-negotiated in the 1970s to specify the number of hours lecturers at various grade should work. The basis for the Audit Commission's Report is the perceived discrepancy between the number of hours colleges are contracted to in terms of staffing levels and the actual number of hours worked in colleges. The Report recommends: an increase in staff–student ratios; that actual class contact hours are monitored to ensure they are within agreed ranges; more lecturer time be spent in class contact so less up-grading of staff; the monitoring of lecturers' use of their out-of-class time to see it is not abused; and the avoidance of over-teaching. Working practices should be renegotiated to get rid of those 'which are not conducive to value for money':

> The reduction in class contact as seniority increases, the lack of minimum class contact hours, teaching years of 33 weeks or less, and timetabling arrangements which permit lecturers to claim overtime payments even though they have not met their contractual hours for the year as a whole, are all aspects of the present arrangements requiring attention. (Audit Commission, 1985: 2).

The concept of professionalism can be used by a profession as 'a strategy for controlling practice' (Esland, 1980: 340) and as a political ploy in the bargaining process over work definition as, for instance, in the profession's claim to 'the organisational corollaries of the independent practitioner' (Green, 1975: 136) in an attempt to protect clinical autonomy. But the use of the notion of professionalism as a device to distance an occupational group from external accountability is increasingly criticized. There is criticism that professionals are no longer actually acting professionally in their attitudes towards contract. In the consultants' contract dispute critics of the consultants' new contract argued that specified hours of work were not appropriate to professional commitments. The Royal Commission described it as 'unprofessional... close to an industrial type of contract in which workers are checked in and out of their place of work and paid for overtime' (Royal Commission, 1975: para 14.67), sentiments echoed in various DDRB reports.

Fox suggests a link between stricter contractual relations and the erosion of trust between employer and employee. Both react to this erosion by moves towards contract. Employers emphasize the obligations of contract, employees its limits. Moves towards contract, by employers or employees, testify to a disequilibrium in the psychological contract. Employees subject to less discretion in their work and closer monitoring react by paying closer attention to the efforts they are willing to devote to it:

> Accustomed to an assumption that they are giving maximum performance in the service of [organizational] ends... they find themselves watched, measured, evaluated, and otherwise regulated by systematic, perhaps even quantitative, criteria. They reciprocate by reducing their commitment [to the organization] and by weighing their contribution in a more calculating spirit. (Fox, 1974: 109)

The excuse of lack of time for not doing certain kinds of work can actually demonstrate a dwindling of commitment (Marks, 1977). A reduction in discretion leads to the alienation of self-estrangement and a diminution in the moral nature of the commitment to work (Fox, 1974: 83). Critics of professionals have discerned precisely this trend (Wilding, 1982). Professionals are not free of the 'calculative expediency' (Fox, 1974: 289) they criticize in others.

Trends towards contract would seem to favour employers and clients rather than professional groups that pursue contracts that are more 'closed'. Moves towards a more work-sensitive, 'closed' contract by professional groups can generate unintended consequences. In further education the contract that was welcomed by lecturers in the 1970s as a major improvement of working conditions in fact opened the door in the 1980s to increased control of those working practices by the use of auditing. Here the concept of 'delinquent community' developed by Crozier (1964) and applied to the medical profession by

Freidson (1975) is useful. Delinquency refers to the rejection of rules imposed on a group and what is construed from outside the group as anomic behaviours. Medical 'delinquency' is not a response to a rigid, authoritarian management system as it was in the case of the French schoolchildren to whom the concept was first applied. It is rather as a reaction to the fear of the possibility of the imposition of such a system that 'delinquency', in the form of the rejection of the legitimacy of outside forces to control professional behaviour, has evolved in the medical profession. A possible unintended consequence of its defensive stance on this issue is that it might hasten the very thing it resists:

> The French schoolchildren were responding to a rigid, authoritarian educational system, but no analogous system, imposed by outsiders, has ever existed for medicine. At best, its delinquent community may be explained by reference to a sense of vulnerability to the possible imposition of such controls: an anticipatory response. The irony is that rather than defending the profession against the imposition of a rigid authority framework, the anticipatory responses of the medical community have created part of the pressure for the institution of such a framework. The failure of the profession to control the availability, cost and quality of the services of its members in the public interest – a failure tied directly to the internal *laissez faire* etiquette of its delinquent community – has contributed to the development ... of externally imposed requirements that may very well come to be, in the future, what the profession has always feared. It may have created what it has anticipated by the very defences it erected. (Freidson, 1975: 246)

By protesting too much the profession, like Hamlet's Queen, might well have alerted the outside world to the possibility that the protests mask, if not guilt, a failure on its part to rationalize and manage its time use according to the problems facing the provision of health care in a situation of resource constraint. The state argues that lack of accountability has led to inefficiency in the provision of services. In medicine stronger line management as advocated by the Griffiths Report (NHS Management Inquiry, 1983) can be interpreted as designed to remove those aspects of the present structure 'which can subvert, resist, or delay central state policies' (Cousins, 1984: 28–30). General managers can side-step consensus management teams, thus short-circuiting the complex NHS consultative machinery which favours medical power over the decision-making process in the NHS. Reaction against consensus management indicates the growth of a new rationality based on the state 'using a model of private capitalistic manufacturing industry when looking for a rational means of controlling a health service' (Manson, 1977: 200). Attempts to introduce precisely such a rationality has been a key aspect of NHS developments in the 1980s. The logic of these developments is that the doctor has to learn that he or she is not an independent practitioner but a member of an organization using finite resources and, ultimately, a servant of the state.

References

Audit Commission for Local Authorities in England and Wales (1985) *Obtaining Better Value for Further Education*. London: HMSO.
Baldamus, W. (1961) *Efficiency and Effort: an analysis of industrial administration*. London: Tavistock.
British Medical Journal (1975) 'Consultant contract discussion', 4 January: 45.
British Medical Journal (1975) 'Consultants contract. Talk about talks come to an end', 22 February: 471.
British Medical Journal (1977) 'Correspondence', 1 January: 53.
British Medical Journal (1979) 'Evidence on new contracts for NHS consultants', 16 June: 1653.
British Medical Journal (1990) 'Letter from Westminster', 3 February: 290.
British Medical Journal (1990) 'Letters from Westminster', 4 August: 225.
Cousins, C. (1984) 'Labour processes in the state service sector', Paper presented to the 2nd Annual Labour Process Conference, Aston University.
Crozier, M. (1964) *The Bureaucratic Phenomenon*. Chicago: Chicago University Press.
Elliott, P. (1975) 'Professional ideology and social situation', in G. Esland, et al. (eds), *People and Work*. Milton Keynes: Open University Press.
Esland, G. (1980) 'Professionals and professionalism', in G. Esland and G. Salaman (eds), *The Politics of Work and Occupation*. Milton Keynes: Open University Press.
Fox, A. (1974) *Beyond Contract: Work, Power and Trust Relations*. London: Faber.
Freidson, E. (1970) *Professional Dominance: the social structure of medical care*. Chicago: Aldine.
Freidson, E. (1975) *Doctoring Together. A study of professional social control*. Chicago: Chicago University Press.
Gordon, H. and Iliffe, S. (1977) *Pickets in White: the junior doctors' dispute of 1975*. London: MPU Publications.
Green, S. (1975) 'Professional/bureaucratic conflict: the case of the medical profession in the NHS', *Sociological Review*, 23: 121–41.
Grossin, W. (1969) *Le travail et le temps. Horaires-durees-rhythmes*. Paris: Eds. Anthropos.
Gurvitch, G. (1963) *The Spectrum of Social Time*. Dordrecht: D. Reidel.
Halmos, P. (ed.) (1973) *Professionalisation and Social Change. Sociological Review Monograph*, no. 20.
Haug, M.R. (1973) 'Deprofessionalization: an alternate hypothesis for the future', in P. Halmos (ed.), *Professionalisation and Social Change. Sociological Review Monograph*, no. 20.
Heydebrand, W.V. (1983) 'Technocratic corporatism. Toward a theory of occupational and organizational transformation', in R.H. Hall and R.E. Quinn (eds), *Organizational Theory and Public Policy*. Beverly Hills: Sage.
House of Commons Social Services Committee (1984) 'Griffiths NHS Management Inquiry Report'. London: HMSO.
Klein, R. (1990) 'The state and the profession: the politics of the double bed', *British Medical Journal*, 301: 700–2.
Lamour, P. and Chalendar, J. (1974) *Prendre le temps de vivre*. Paris: le Seuil.

Manson, T. (1977) 'Management, the professions and the unions: a social analysis of change in the National Health Service', in M. Stacey et al. (eds), *Health and the Division of Labour*. London: Croom Helm.

Marks, S.R. (1977) 'Multiple roles and role strain: some notes on human energy, time and commitment', *American Sociological Review*, 42: 921–36.

Mumford, L. (1973) *Interpretations and Forecasts*. New York: Harcourt, Brace, Jovanovich.

NHS Management Inquiry (1983) 'Report' [the Griffiths Report]. London: DHSS.

O'Connor, J. (1972) *The Fiscal Crisis of the State*. New York: St. Martin's Press.

Review Body on Doctors' and Dentists' Remuneration (DDRB) (1977) *Seventh Report*. London: HMSO.

Review Body on Doctors' and Dentists' Remuneration (DDRB) (1978) *Eighth Report*. London: HMSO.

Royal Commission on the National Health Service (1979) *Report*. London: HMSO.

Secretaries of State for Health (1989) *Working for Patients*. London: HMSO.

Starkey, K.P. (1986) 'Time and Professional Work in Public Sector Organisations'. Unpublished PhD thesis, Aston University.

Thompson, E.P. (1967) 'Time, work-discipline and industrial capitalism', *Past and Present*. 36: 57–97.

Weber, M. (1976) *The Protestant Ethic and the Spirit of Capitalism*. London: Allen and Unwin.

Wilding, P. (1982) *Professional Power and Social Welfare*. London: Routledge and Kegan Paul.

Zerubavel, E. (1981) *Hidden Rhythms: Schedules and calendars in social life*. Chicago: Chicago University Press.

7

Broken Rhythms and Unmet Deadlines: workers' and managers' time-perspectives

Paul Bellaby

> To begin with, the fact of illness means an interruption in the rhythm of...life.... The beginning and the end of daily work, the hours of meals, all these make up the rhythm of our lives, which vibrates in a different tempo for city dweller, for farmer, for factory worker, for white collar worker.
> .... An undisturbed rhythm means health. A change in that rhythm, perhaps when a farmer moves into the city and starts a city job, means a risk to health and produces altered conditions of illness and treatment. (Sigerist 1929/1977: 389)

Giddens (1979, 1984) points out that mainstream (functionalist) sociology has conflated time with change. His object, like mine here, is to show that attending to time in social action is just as important when the same thing happens over and again. I also want to avoid the merely programmatic and give a substantive account of how workers and managers usually sustain effort at work and occasionally go sick.

Social processes unfold in time. As in a juggling act, structure has to be worked at – in this sense, the balls have to be kept in the air no less when the same juggling routine is repeated than when it is changed for a new one. However, the time in which social processes unfold is itself a social construct.

The clock and calendar times familiar in the modern world are built upon principles, some of which are in nature, but many of which, such as the week, are conventional. The division of the day and night, regardless of season and of latitude, into 24 hours, 24×60 minutes and 24×60 seconds is arbitrary in Saussure's sense (1916/1974: 67–70). Shared time, however measured, is thus closer to language than to nature. In particular, clock and calendar are typical of the spatial metaphors by which time is depicted in Western culture (Fabian, 1983). However, the use of spatial metaphors applies rather to the language of (pre-twentieth century) physical science and of most social science (up to our own time), than to everyday practice. Traditionally in the West at least, time has been experienced in two frames: the first linear and irreversible – in relation to one's own life course; and the second cyclical and repetitive – in relation to darkness and light, the seasons and succession of generations. In neither form is time measured out in standard lengths.

Standardization began under the seventh-century monastic rule of St Benedict of Nursia (Zerubavel, 1981: chapter 2). The hora divided day and night without regard to darkness and light. For instance, monks were disciplined to rise from their beds at dead of night to celebrate the office. This was partly because obedience was an end in itself in monastic observance, partly because 'batch-living' necessitated a common timetable (Roth 1963; Goffman 1968). This disciplinary aspect of time within organizations forms the link between Sigerist's observations on health and the study of sickness absence at work. For, following in the footsteps of monasticism, the nineteenth-century railway network (McKenna 1980) and (later than Thompson (1967) suggests) bureaucratized factory work, required time discipline of employees and/or customers. If the purpose was now more instrumental than moral, the degree of acquiescence required of the subject was scarcely less than had been the case in monastic life.

The discipline of clock and calendar has come to be normalized with the growth of towns and industry and commerce – that is to say, to be seen as a fact of nature, rather than of social convention. Time discipline, no less than the spatial distribution of populations under surveillance that Foucault (1975/1977) has explored, is inextricable from power. This is brought out by McKenna (1980) in his history of British railwaymen. From the development of regional, then national networks (from the 1840s), punctuality to uniform national time became the *raison d'être* of railway management, and placed power in the hands of those who made and administered timetables, and even of the driver, who, unlike the fireman, was issued with a pocket watch.

Power is relational. It can scarcely be said to be the possession of one person or group, but flows within relations as one party seeks control and the other resists. This insight, currently attributed to Foucault (1977/1979, 1982), is by no means new to industrial sociology. The literature is full of examples of individual workers and work groups resisting management. A specific form this takes is making time for oneself in the working day (Roethlisberger and Dickson, 1934; Roy 1959; Lupton 1968). I suggest that going sick at work is a special case of making time for oneself. It is distinguished from others by the fact that sickness, if successfully negotiated, can claim the sympathy and indulgence of others (on this ambiguity, and the play it gives to employees, see Bellaby 1990).

Going sick contains at least two phases. The second phase, which has been studied far more often than the first, is that of diagnosis, treatment and discharge/death. Even here, Strauss et al. (1985) show how in hospital acute episodes of chronic diseases take on a trajectory dictated by the timescales of medical technology and organization, rather than by the biological features of the diseases themselves. I focus on the first phase of the sickness process. This is effectively prehistory, because it is rarely documented by health workers, far less often than the other, and we must rely either on direct observation by ethnographers or (auto)biography to establish what happens.[1]

Time at work: external and internal, linear and cyclical

There are fruitful analogies between how time is experienced in everyday work and how the time of a long journey may be experienced. Canto-Klein (1975) has followed Proust's (1921/1941) example and analysed subjective time on long train journeys, but in her case with the aid of a social survey commissioned by the French railways. The passenger has no control over the external time that elapses between stations; and there is time to fill that is internal to the train: 'il faut "occuper le temps", "passer le temps", "tuer le temps", "vaincre la monotonie du voyage"' (Canto-Klein, 1975: 364). First and second class and regular, as opposed to occasional, first class travellers differ in the pastimes they choose.

A similar 'class' difference is to be found between managers and workers in a pottery factory. It is attributable largely to the different facilities available to each for passing the time. Zerubavel (1979) has shown that organizations typically give higher grade personnel more flexibility in use of time and space than their subordinates. The manager can vary his or her activity, pause in the middle of an operation, and escape from surveillance into an office. Some workers (for example, craft workers and warehouse labourers) have some of these facilities, legitimately or not, but most (especially machine attendants and assembly line operatives) have their work-pace and spells of activity determined for them, and work in full view of managers and other workers (Bellaby, 1986). This is one of the givens of internal time, that time which both managers and workers must occupy within the work period, rather than external time which they divide between employment on the one hand and leisure (or work) at home or in the community.

Another given is the predominantly linear or cyclical character with which time presents itself, and this too differs for managers and workers. There is no equivalent to this aspect of time in the railway journey. For semi-skilled workers, especially on machine- or line-paced work, the cyclical aspect dominates the linear. Linear time is typically broken down into units of different length: spells between breaks, the shift, the five day week, intervals between holidays, and ultimately the working life itself. Within each of these categories, units are of the same length. Thus, linear time takes on a largely cyclical aspect: one day is much like another, week succeeds week; and the cycles resemble economic cycles of varying length, the longer over-arching the shorter (Braudel 1979/1984: 71–88; cf. Bellaby (1989) on cyclical patterns of absence from work).

Managers too have quite regular work schedules, more so than academics (and perhaps Yuppies – Barr and York (1987)), but less so by far than those they manage. Indeed, the schedules become less regular, the higher the manager is on the career ladder on which he started. The Vice-Chairman of the company said he felt entitled to a round of golf on a working day every now and then, because he frequently worked late at the office or took work home. Not only is this cyclical aspect of work blurred in the case of managers, the linear aspect is accentuated. Time tends to be divided into unequal lengths which correspond to assignments – batches to be produced, new products to be brought on stream, a marketing campaign to be brought to fruition and evaluated. Instead of these lengths being laid end to end (one day after another, and so on), they often overlap, such that one is beginning while another ends and a third continues. Moreover, managers have 'careers': they usually aspire to be at certain points on a ladder by specific ages. In that sense, their working life itself is linear, not merely part of a life cycle shared with other members of the group of family and kin.

Unlike internal time, external time presents itself to traveller and industrial employee alike as that which can be altered only by ceasing to be present, by not boarding the train, by absenting oneself from work. However, absence may be a response to what becomes, for many possible reasons, insuperable difficulty in negotiating time internal to work. Both managers and workers have to present a front of sustained effort to superiors, and not least to peers and subordinates. The limited facilities available to semi-skilled workers in mechanized or flow-designed production make it hard for them to fool their managers. They have to sustain effort (rather than an appearance of effort). How are they able to do so?

Rhythm

Donald Roy, who perhaps pioneered participant observation of mech-anized factory work, laid stress on the pastimes that individuals and work groups devised to while away the hours and counter the monotony (Roy, 1954). Without denying the relevance of this, I suggest that what makes it possible to turn work into a game, to daydream while working or to soldier on grimly – whatever one's personal adaptation, is rhythm.

> The line ran more smoothly than yesterday and I tried hard to feed the ware through with the right gaps. By mid-morning I was feeding more or less automatically and was able to attend to things around me a little. I felt far less fatigued at the end of the day, in spite of the pressure of work. (Field notes taken when learning to feed a moving line that sprayed glaze on tableware.)

According to Marx (1867/1976: Parts 3 and 4), as capitalism developed, time in work was successively lengthened to increase production and shortened as productivity was increased. In both phases of development, industry has periodically disrupted rhythms: at first, those of darkness and light and the seasons that enfold the life and work of peasants no less tyrannically than the clock, but differently; and, latterly, rhythmic patterns which have been steadily remade by workers after each wave of technological and organizational change. Moreover, workers' rhythm is both synergistic with the disciplines that work and its organization have imposed, and in conflict with capital's principle of economy of labour-time.

The pottery industry of North Staffs has seen such a pattern of workers establishing rhythm at the heart of workplace culture and relations, and economic and technical change breaking in to disrupt that rhythm, since the late-eighteenth century. Potters, notably Josiah Wedgwood, are credited with early innovation in the division of labour and production management (McKendrick, 1961). However, as Samuel (1977) has shown, most forms of work, here as elsewhere in British industry, remained manual, rather than becoming mechanized, until well into this century (see also Pollard (1968) on the slow development of bureaucratic management and its reflection in Shaw's (1903/1969) autobiographical account of pottery work in the nineteenth century). Since the major reorganizations following the Second World War (Gay and Smith, 1974), the pottery industry has been rather rapidly converted to near-flow production and mechanization, and has already ventured into automation (Till, 1987). By itself, change breaks rhythms in manual work. But making the potter's arm and wrist an adjunct to a machine and moving line, presents further possibilities of disruption of rhythm due both to mechanical failures and to the non-variable pace of moving lines.

Mechanization of this degree has been associated in the pottery industry, as in electrical and electronic assembly work, with a virtual epidemic of repetition strain injuries (RSI) in the last decade (known more widely, though imprecisely as 'tenosynovitis' or 'teno' for short) (Thompson et al., 1987). The apparent epidemic is partly political in cause, here as in Australia (Bennett, 1985): in North Staffordshire it is known among both personnel managers and union officials as a 'bandwagon', the number of applicants for compensation having risen sharply after a successful claim against the large Wedgwood group in 1986. RSI is probably linked with how work is organized: its pace, the provision of rest pauses, abrupt changes (including return to a familiar job after an absence), and interpersonal relations (Thompson et al., 1987: 83). In what follows I wish to suggest that RSI is a special case of many injuries and much sickness that arise from the kind of repetition that breaks rhythm or makes it difficult to achieve rhythm.

How rhythm is established in manual work
There has been much attention to biological rhythms in the literature on work: in particular, to the relation between the circadian (daily) inbuilt clock and patterns of shift work (Reinberg et al., 1984; Waterhouse et al., 1987). In the present context, circadian rhythms have little relevance. To sustain repetitive manual labour, it is plain that each individual must find his or her own rhythm, and that biology constrains or enables peripherally at best. Nor is that rhythm altogether idiosyncratic. Rather it is social and cultural, even though in the pottery factory workers do not usually work rhythmically in unison. An established rhythm for a given job is a property of the workplace and often of generations who have worked there. It is taught to novices by experienced workers. For instance, when, in the second of the two jobs I did on the shopfloor (kiln-emptying), I began lifting loads of around 15 kilos off a roller-conveyor repeatedly through the day, I was told by my experienced mate not to 'maul', that is to pull loads towards me, but to allow them to fall gently onto my outstretched arms, which, of course, saved considerable muscular wear and tear. Similarly those who print patterns onto mugs by machine move their whole bodies to reach mugs from pallets to their right, apply the print and then place them on pallets to their left, in a pendulum like motion. This minimizes back strain. In general, workers may use pop music on the tannoy or singing to help sustain rhythm.

As Laban and his followers understood, dance is a useful analogy for the way manual work is performed to rhythm (Laban and Lawrence, 1947; Maletic, 1987). Each job has its unwritten choreography. This has two components of particular interest: beat and phrasing. Beat is not given by machinery, it is worked out by actors within the constraints of machinery and workflow. Phrasing is the equivalent of a sequence of steps. The scheduling of work provides for the development of phrasing. Phrasing does not necessarily coincide with breaks the management makes in the working day, with the week or the intervals between holidays, as Muslim workers in the potbank make most obvious, for of course British working hours cut across Islamic religious festivals, Friday prayers and daily times of prayer.

My fellow kiln emptiers imposed the discipline of an autonomous work-group (cf. Trist et al., 1963) upon the beat and phrasing of members. Most members of the team had worked together for at least 15 years, and they spoke of how, in the face of many threats of disruption by management, they had steadily evolved a (very fast) beat, and a phrasing that permitted an early finish with only one break during the shift. So finely tuned were individuals to the collective rhythm that one of my mates complained of muscular pains and a headache when a supply failure carried our work well over the usual finish time, and another showed how he had lacerated his hands on the rough structure of a kiln truck by setting himself fractionally out of position as he began work.

Workers who, unlike these men, had lost within their working lives a traditional rhythm, experienced this as (in effect) loss of autonomy: an instance is casters (usually male) and spongers (usually female), who in one workshop, have been obliged to work set hours regardless of whether they complete what they see to be their quota for the day, and who find even the enforced breakfast and lunch breaks disruptive.

Broken rhythm and absence from work

The process of going sick in manual work is often connected intrinsically with broken rhythm. It accounts for fatigue and fatigue feeds back upon it. Taking time off is a way of recovering the means to get back into step.

Taylorist job design tends to remove two sources of rhythm in manual work: the leeway to work at one's own pace and the redundancy in motion by which people might communicate to each other a shared rhythm. We set up in the pottery factory job-redesign experiments on Taylorized and mechanized production lines (Bellaby, 1985). Workers on these lines were almost all women. Typically, women do more of the jobs in which use of time (and space) is restricted than do men. It is also the case that the ratio of managers and supervisors to operatives is usually higher in such jobs.

One of the three experiments was essentially a production engineering change, involving the removal of part of the process from the moving line. Since this had been a breakdown bottleneck, the line now worked less discontinuously, and so put 'pressure' (in the women's words) on workers still on the line. In the first six weeks or so, there was a sharp rise in losses in the course of production (which averaged 11.3 per cent of throughput in the first month) and in sickness absence (which reached an average of 25 per cent per day in the second month). However, when workers found a means of re-establishing pauses, and thus phrasing, by rotating jobs among themselves, there was a marked recovery in both losses (which fell progressively to 4.7 per cent of throughput in the fifth month) and sickness absence (which fell sharply to 6.4 per cent per day by the fifth month).

Another experiment involved the addition of a worker whose sole responsibility was to relieve women on the line as and when they asked. This displaced a system in which the supervisor relieved workers at two times in the day by rotation and for no more than five minutes. The new system reduced absence by comparison with the corresponding period in the previous year (from 6.3 per cent to 5.2 per cent per day) and pushed losses down (from 6.6 per cent to 5.2 per cent of throughput): a third fewer faults over target were found at the daily sample dissections than was the norm for the department (1.31 on average on this line, as compared with 1.98 to 2.19 on three others). The women emphasized not only that the relief worker allowed them as much rest when they needed it as was appropriate to their feelings on the day, but also that their sense of team work was reinforced. In other words, collective rhythm could now be reasserted in conditions otherwise disruptive to it.

However, the largest fall in sickness absence occurred on the third experimental production line, where (at the women's suggestion) the finish time on Friday was brought forward from 3.30 pm to 12.30 pm, in exchange for an earlier start each day. Here absence averaged 3 per cent over the experimental period, and was as low as 1 per cent by the fifth month. Someone said that they had gained a four and a half day working week and a two and a half day weekend. Thus the change affected women's time-budgets. As it happens, none had still dependent children, but – whether single or married – they felt that the 'free' Friday afternoon made time for leisure at the weekend by allowing them to bring shopping and housework forward. This change in external time (or time elapsing while inside the factory) was paralleled by change in internal time. The end of the week, participants said, was brought forward, so that by the middle of the week, with Thursday pay day to look forward to and a short spell on Friday, they felt less fatigued than normally.

Broken rhythm and the sick role
Of course, it remains possible for individuals to find difficulty in matching their workmates' rhythm, and so to experience anxiety and fatigue while others are on good form. In the group of kiln emptiers with whom I worked, occasional lapses in performance and also the pains of learning the job, were accommodated by others making up: they had to be or the group would be unable to achieve its quota of work and leave at its chosen time. One member, however, had

persistent difficulty in keeping up with the others. He came in fifteen or more minutes early and worked on at breakfast and when others finished at lunch, in order to empty his share of kiln trucks.

> Events of the day were overshadowed by Bill having an epileptic seizure. It was not allowed to interfere with the pace of work to any great extent. He had a premonitory 'tremor' again before breakfast (several last week). Then after breakfast he was sitting on the rollers with Sam by him. The manager was passing through and was asked to come quickly. Bill was now standing, held on either side and convulsing, his eyes apparently closed. The manager, with difficulty, removed Bill's teeth. Tom (as safety rep) was called on and also Gladys (first aid). A blanket and a pillow were brought and Bill was carried from the line and laid out, covered over. Gladys was left by him.
>
> Sam felt management should recognise that Bill was a danger to himself and to others and should be taken off the job. It was the stress of catching up that had brought the fits on. He had raised his four kids, and no longer needed the big money.

As the above excerpts from field notes show, Bill's epilepsy was common knowledge in the workplace, and others were quite adept at handling his seizures, and by no means unsympathetic to him. Even so, his normally well-controlled epilepsy was becoming a disability. This is largely because it was defined as such by his fellow workers (more so than by his manager) and because increasingly Bill was acceding to this label. The individual example illustrates not only that rhythm is a social product, part of workplace culture, which is transmitted by the group and reinforced by interaction, but that evidence of broken rhythm is so reacted to by workmates that the victim may be impelled towards the sick role.

It is tempting to romance about rhythm in manual work, much as Braverman (1974) has about skill, but with the opposite effect, namely of suggesting that semi-skilled workers accommodate readily to the demands of fragmented and repetitive wage labour. The example of Bill helps show how rhythm may pose problems for workers rather than solve them. It should also be pointed out that rhythm does not remove all the physical strains and deadening monotony of Taylorized work.

Deadlines

On the whole, managers' performance is less visible than that of shopfloor workers. Crucially, it is made visible to superiors by the imposition of deadlines by which certain tasks have to be completed. Managers are made to account for their achievement, which as often as not depends on that of their subordinates. Sometimes deadlines are frequent and specific. The lowest level of departmental manager in the potbank has production targets to meet each week, which include levels of waste and of quality control. The next level of management is responsible for budgeting for consumables on a monthly basis. In Jaques's (1982) terms, each has his or her own 'time-span of discretion'. Alternatively, deadlines occur at regular but infrequent intervals throughout managers' careers and are the points at which they are judged ripe for promotion, or unlikely to be able to carry greater responsibility.

A corollary of control by deadlines is that what at first appears to be managers' greater freedom to use time at work, turns out to be the right of superiors to invade their informal time – in the canteen, the washroom and the corridor, often also at home. In potbanks the kiln manager may be permanently on call, because kilns are only shut down during the Potters' Holidays. Managers also take work home. The right of the firm to call for this commitment is symbolized by the fact that overtime payment is usually denied to staff above the lowest levels. It is of course paid routinely to shopfloor workers. Middle managers, who are in a grey area from this point of view, often prove aware that to press for overtime payment is to risk being defined as one who lacks the 'right attitude' for management.

Managers are encouraged to view their future with the company in individual terms. Rather than adopting the (steady) rhythm of the experienced managers, new recruits should seek to outpace their peers. In spite of a public grade system, salary levels and fringe benefits vary widely on the same grade. Managers we interviewed could not guess the earnings of their peers in the same company. Each, it seems, was the beneficiary of patronage by a superior, or else victim of its withdrawal. Managerial structure was not so much a bureaucracy: rather it was patrimonial (Weber 1925/1968: 217–37).

Managers' time off for sickness is treated flexibly by the company. A sick manager does not lose earnings until at least three months' absence; whereas a sick manual worker loses some of his or her earnings even while the company sick pay scheme applies (the first two months) and thereafter must apply for social security payments. However, the flexibility conceals the assumption that a manager will take sick leave 'responsibly' (on the concept of 'responsible autonomy', but not its underside, see Friedman, 1977). Prolonged or frequent absence, even through sickness, is taken to call in question a manager's ability to meet deadlines. Significantly, managers defend themselves by attributing their sick leave to disease or injury that arises from stress. They are also aware that such a defence calls in question their capacity to cope with their jobs, since a good manager can handle the pressure.

These generalizations can be illustrated by a case study of the social relation between four managers (all, as is typical, male), who are in direct line of command: Charles the managing director, Nigel the production director, Bob the second tier manager, and Jack the departmental manager.

The managing director has a private income and (financially) does not have a great deal to lose by retiring and giving up his salary, though it allows him to support his sons' private education and he says that it gives him the satisfaction of not being a 'parasite'. The other men are career managers, Nigel and Bob having reached managerial status before they joined the firm, but Jack having been promoted first to supervisor, then to departmental manager from the shopfloor. They work in a unit which is beleaguered by poor sales performance.

'Stress' is on the lips, or at least the tip-of-the-tongue of Nigel, Bob and Jack in discussing their work and their health:

Nigel: In the last two weeks I have felt more tired than usual. The pressure of the business has changed so much. I am under pressure to turn the business round, and under fierce attack from Charles. Charles has acted on a customer's complaint by turning the aggro on individuals. I was never consulted ... The downside to this job is the way the human relations aspect is handled. There should be more forward planning. Mistakes are bound to be made. Then individuals are blamed. People are got down by it. [On being asked whether he was given sufficient control to do his job properly, laughing] I decided a long time ago, it is easier to become a 'yes' man. So 'yes'. I am given the authority. I carry the responsibility. But make a mistake and you are dealt with severely.

Bob: Over the year, my health has deteriorated because of my job. I suffer from chronic muscular tension. The doctor puts it down to stress. Fifteen months ago it reached its peak. I was not delegating: I was prepared to take all the stress on my own shoulders ... I find it frustrating that the established workforce do not accept that we mean to make things better – there is mistrust, they suspect any change as a management tool. It is also frustrating seeing things not going right, and that you could jump in and solve it. But I have to leave subordinates to do the job.

Jack: [All four men said they enjoyed 'responsibility'] I admit I enjoy responsibility. In management as opposed to the shopfloor I bring in the word 'involvement'. I enjoy seeing something coming together, fulfilling a plan on a daily, no more a weekly basis: good counts and quality. [On being asked about the bad side of the job] How long have you got? Pressure – an awful lot. Can be a tremendous mental strain. A manager, unlike an operative, is always on trial, always got to be 100 per cent committed. You take the knocks for other people's lack of interest. We get the rough side of [superiors'] tongues, a dogmatic approach. Sometimes I wonder if the financial rewards are worth it. Other people come in and change things I have set up. You're the bad guy, you get the backlash from the [shopfloor] people and from senior managers and the director.

The three men in the beleaguered unit all personalize stress: both its source, which in more or less veiled manner is seen to be each person's immediate superior and often a mistrustful workforce, and their responsibility to handle stress – Bob says he has had to learn to delegate; Nigel hints at diplomatic manoeuvres, learning to be a 'yes-man'. The managing director is, of course, the immediate (though not the sole) source of the pressure upon the production director, a pressure which is transferred, as in Newton's cradle, along the line of command to the point at which Bob and to a greater extent Jack experience the cross-pressures of 'men in the middle', between top management and shopfloor.

Conclusion

Health at work is an adaptation to the time constraints that accompany the organization of work. Speaking broadly, semi-skilled manual work and line management involve different patterns of time internal to work. In the manual jobs, cyclical aspects dominate linear aspects; in the managerial, linear aspects dominate the cyclical aspects. Adaptation to the two patterns is learned from others. Workers acquire rhythm and managers a capacity to balance assignments and fulfil the deadlines they impose.

Sickness and injury arise when the adaptations fail. Taking time off is to break step with work in the hope of recovering rhythm later; or legitimately to evade current deadlines in order to gain control over future assignments. Managers more often have the facilities to avoid time off by taking a rest-pause in the course of work itself than do semi-skilled workers.

Managers experience 'stress' when their adaptation is failing, but also attribute the failure to loss of control or 'coping' ability on their part. This explanation has been given general currency in many accounts of sickness, injury and absence. But it should be treated with caution. First, it erases the important difference I have demonstrated between the time constraints and adaptations found in manual and managerial jobs. Second, stress and coping discourse is rooted in managerial experience, but is also a class ideology. It may be used by managers and professionals to underline the 'mental' (as opposed to physical) demands of their type of work (cf. Bendix, 1956/1963). More significantly, it is the ideology by which the employer controls his or her agents – the managers themselves (cf. Young, 1980).

Until the present recession, sickness absence had risen year by year in Britain from the Second World War (Bellaby, et al., 1984). The British Ceramic Manufacturers' Federation was not alone in seeing it as a major threat to productive efficiency, losing as it did some twenty times as many working days as disputes, even in the 1960s. If our work in the pottery industry can be generalized, then disruption to work rhythms as a result of managerial rationalization and mechanization of production has a large share of responsibility. The counterpart for the growing army of managers has been inter-polation of several tiers in any line of command and the practice of giving each manager a sphere of jurisdiction, for which, nevertheless, he or she was regularly accountable to superiors. It cannot be over-looked that the academics who have elaborated the 'stress and coping' representation of the bureaucratic demiurge, have themselves become subject to deadlines and all that goes with them.

Even in the case of managers we should not mistake an ideology which is the product of the manager's situation for the underlying cause. 'Going sick' must first and foremost be understood as a culturally embedded social process (Frankenberg, 1986), the di-mensions of which are shared with the organization of work itself. Mapping time as one of those dimensions has illustrated that broader argument.

Notes

I am indebted to my former colleagues at Keele University and especially to Judith Sidaway and Sheila Cleverly; also to the directors, employees and trade unions at Staffordshire Potteries Ltd. The research project was funded by two grants from the Economic and Social Research Council (for Final Reports, see Bellaby, 1985, 1987), and latterly by Staffordshire Potteries itself. I am grateful for comments on earlier versions of this chapter from Barbara Adam, Mel Bartley, Mick Bloor, Gibson Burrell, Ronnie Frankenberg, Marion McLeod, Sylvia Shimin, Judith Sidaway, David Vincent and Tony Williams.

1. In the present study of a pottery factory employing 800 in tableware manufacture, fieldwork included: two investigators doing participant observation as full-time labourers with four contrasted work groups for six months; the completion of two-week diaries by those we had worked with on the shopfloor; interviews with a stratified random sample of 200 production workers and a sample of 50 managerial and supervisory staff, including directors in the line of command; and the collection of retrospective absence, sickness and other personnel records for three years of the two samples and the four work-groups. Later we collaborated with the company and some of its (women) workers and managers in changing the way in which work was organized and monitoring the effects on sickness absence and productivity (Bellaby, 1985, 1987).

References

Barr, Ann and York, Peter (1987) 'The new Babylon: just the job', *The Observer*, Review, 8 November: 21–2.
Bellaby, P. (1985) *Experiments in Changing Work Organization at Staffordshire Potteries Ltd.* London: Economic and Social Research Council.
Bellaby, P. (1986) '"Please boss, can I leave the line?" A sociological alternative to

stress and coping in explaining sickness and absence at work', in B. Judkins (ed.), *Occupational Health, International Journal of Sociology and Social Policy*, 6(4): 52–68.

Bellaby, P. (1987) *The Relation between Work Organization and Sickness Absence in the Pottery Industry*. London: Economic and Social Research Council.

Bellaby, P. (1989) 'The social meanings of time off work: a case study from a pottery factory', *Annals of Occupational Hygiene*, 33: 423–38.

Bellaby, P. (1990) 'What is a genuine sickness? The relation between work discipline and the sick role in a pottery factory', *Sociology of Health and Illness*, 12: 47–68.

Bellaby, P., Cleverly, S. and Sidaway, J.E. (1984) 'The recession and the effort bargain', paper read to the *British Sociological Association*, Annual Conference, Bradford University.

Bendix, R. (1956/1963) *Work and Authority in Industry*. New York: Harper Torchbooks.

Bennett, M.J. (1985) 'The politics of repetitive strain injury', *The Journal of Occupational Health and Safety Australia and New Zealand*, 1: 102–5.

Braudel, F. (1979/1984) *Civilization and Capitalism*, Vol. 3 (The Perspective of the World), translated by Sian Reynolds. London: Collins.

Braverman, H. (1974) *Labor and Monopoly Capital*. New York: Monthly Review Press.

Canto-Klein, M. (1975) 'La réprésentation de l'éspace et du temps: étude sur un type de voyage en chemin de fer', *Cahiers Internationaux de Sociologie*, 59: 355–66.

Fabian, J. (1983) *Time and the Other*. New York: Columbia University Press.

Foucault, M. (1975/1977) *Discipline and Punish*, translated by A.M. Sheridan. Harmondsworth: Allen Lane.

Foucault, M. (1977/1979) *The History of Sexuality*, Vol. 1 (Introduction), translated by A.M. Sheridan. Harmondsworth: Penguin.

Foucault, M. (1982) 'The subject, knowledge and power', in H.L. Dreyfuss and P. Rabinow (eds), *Michel Foucault: Beyond Structuralism and Hermeneutics*. London: Harvester. pp. 208–26.

Frankenberg, R.J. (1986) 'Sickness as cultural performance: drama, trajectory and pilgrimage root metaphors and the making of disease', *International Journal of Health Services*, 16(4): 603–26.

Friedman, A. (1977) *Industry and Labour*. London: Macmillan.

Gay, P.W. and Smith, R.L. (1974) *The British Pottery Industry*. London: Butterworth.

Giddens, A. (1979) *Central Problems in Social Theory*. London: Macmillan.

Giddens, A. (1984) *The Constitution of Society: Outline of a Theory of Structuration*. Cambridge: Polity Press.

Goffman, E. (1968) *Asylums: Essays on the Social Situation of Mental Patients and other Inmates*. Harmondsworth: Penguin.

Jaques, E. (1982) *The Forms of Time*. London: Heinemann.

Laban, R. and Lawrence, F.C. (1947) *Effort*. London: McDonald and Evans.

Lupton, T. (1968) 'Beyond PBR?', in D. Pym (ed.), *Industrial Society*, Harmondsworth: Penguin. pp. 294–315.

Maletic, V. (1987) *Body – Space – Expression: the Development of Rudolf Laban's Movement and Dance Concepts*. Berlin: Mouton de Gruyter.

Marx, K. (1867/1976) *Capital*, Vol. 1, translated by B. Fowkes. Harmondsworth: Penguin.

McKendrick, N. (1961) 'Josiah Wedgwood and factory discipline', *Historical Journal*, 4(1): 30–55.

McKenna, F. (1980) *The Railway Workers 1840–1970*. London: Faber.

Pollard, S. (1968) *The Genesis of Modern Management*. Harmondsworth: Penguin.

Proust, M. (1921/1941) *Cities of the Plain*, Part 2, translated by C.K. Scott-Moncrieff. London: Chatto and Windus.

Reinberg, A., Andlauer, P., De Prins, J., Malbecq, W., Vieux, N. and Laporte, A. (1984) 'Desynchronisation of the oral temperature circadian rhythm and intolerance to shift work', *Nature*, 308 (5956): 272–4.

Roethlisberger, R.J. and Dickson, W.J. (1934) *Management and the Worker*. Cambridge, Mass.: Harvard University Press.

Roth, J. (1963) *Timetables: Structuring the Passage of Time in Hospital Treatment and Other Careers*. New York: Bobbs-Merrill.

Roy, D. (1959) ' "Banana time", job satisfaction and informal interaction', *Human Organization*, 18(4): 158–68.

Samuel, R. (1977) 'Workshop of the world', *History Workshop*, 3: 6–72.

Saussure, F. (1916/1974) *Course in General Linguistics*, translated by W. Baskin. London: Fontana.

Shaw, C. (1903/1969) *When I was a Child*. London: S.R. Publishers.

Sigerist, H. (1929/1977) in D. Landy (ed.) *Culture, Disease and Healing*. London: Collier Macmillan.

Strauss, A., Fagerhaugh, S., Suczek, B. and Wiener, C. (1985) *The Social Organization of Medical Work*. Chicago: Chicago University Press.

Thompson, D., Rawlings, A.J. and Harrington, J.M. (1987) 'Repetition strain injuries', in J.M. Harrington (ed.), *Recent Advances in Occupational Health*, Vol. 3. Edinburgh: Churchill Livingstone.

Thompson, E.P. (1967) 'Time, work-discipline and industrial capitalism', *Past and Present*, 36: 57–97.

Till, A. (1987) 'New tableware production methods', paper read to the *Joint Symposium on Health and Safety in the Ceramics Industry*, British Occupational Health Society and North Staffordshire Medical Institute (Arlidge Section), Stoke on Trent.

Trist, E.L., Higgins, G.W., Murray, H. and Pollock, A.B. (1963) *Organizational Choice*. London: Tavistock.

Waterhouse, J.M., Minors, D.S. and Scott, A.R. (1987) 'Circadian rhythms, intercontinental travel and shift work', in W. Gardner (ed.), *Occupational Health*, Vol. 3. London: Wright.

Weber, M. (1925/1968) *Economy and Society*, Vol. 1, translated by G. Roth and C. Wittich. New York: Bedminster Press.

Young, A. (1980) 'The discourse on stress and the reproduction of conventional knowledge', *Social Science and Medicine*, 14B(3): 133–46.

Zerubavel, E. (1979) *Patterns of Time in Hospital Life: A Sociological Perspective*. Chicago: Chicago University Press.

Zerubavel, E. (1981) *Hidden Rhythms: Schedules and calendars in social life*. Chicago: Chicago University Press.

8

Work, Time and Sickness in the Lives of Schoolchildren

Alan Prout

Bellaby (1992; see Chapter 7) has suggested that the process of sickness contains at least two phases. The second of these (diagnosis, treatment and discharge/death) has formed the main focus of study for anthropologists and sociologists while the first phase, 'going sick', is in his words 'effectively prehistory, because it is rarely documented by health workers' (1992: 109–10), or, one might add, social scientists. The study which Bellaby and his colleagues carried out in an English pottery factory has begun to explore this less familiar territory, piecing together an ethnography of going sick at work. Their work suggests, inter alia, that two socially constructed phenomena, work and time, are crucially implicated in the process. In particular they delineate a dual aspect to the temporal organization of work: 'rhythm' and 'deadline'. They propose that '. . . [sickness] occurs either when rhythm is broken or when deadlines cannot be met. Then individuals seek to make time for themselves by pleading sickness and others may permit them to fall out of step or postpone the deadline' (ibid.).

In this chapter I will examine some of the ways in which the social organization of time and work were related to going sick among a class of English primary schoolchildren. My analysis is based on fieldwork material drawn from a wider ethnographic study of sickness absence in an English primary school (see also Prout, 1986, 1987). It is necessary first to indicate some of my theoretical and methodological starting points. The basic issues will be familiar to those who have followed recent writing on the sociology and anthropology of childhood (see James and Prout, 1990). A central concern of these recent discussions and of this chapter has been the recognition of children as interpretive social actors. This is a departure from 'socialization', for so long the dominant concept for the analysis of childhood, but now seen as problematic since it tends to construct children as passive, incompetent and asocial beings.

Fieldwork and setting[1]

The empirical material on which this chapter is based was gathered between March and July of 1982 in a small primary school, which I have called 'Appletrees'. The school was located in a semi-suburban village on the outskirts of an English city. Like most English primary schools, Appletrees taught children between the ages of 7 and 11 who were organized into four 'year' groups. Each 'year' was divided into two 'forms' who were taught by a separate teacher. I focused most of my attention on one of these forms, 4F, which comprised the oldest children in the school. The class consisted of 35 children, equally divided between boys and girls, and their teacher, Catherine Frazer. All the children were due to move on to the next stage within the English schooling system ('secondary school') at the start of the next academic year, in September. Most of the children were scheduled to go to a nearby co-educational comprehensive school which I have called 'Lowhouse'. This school separated the children into different 'ability bands' on the basis of the children's performance in a series of examinations which the children sat during the last term of their primary schooling.

The study was small scale, intensive and processual (Gluckman, 1961; Mitchell, 1983). I followed up every case of sickness absence among the children of 4F over the summer term, gathering material in interviews with the children, parents and teachers, through observation in the school, and through health diaries that various informants kept over the period. I also had access to the school attendance register. The whole range of this material will be drawn upon in the analysis which follows.

Children's participation in the process of sickness

Although there are occasions when children are declared sick by adults and have no active part in the process, this is not the situation with the bulk of their everyday sicknesses (that is, the acute non-life threatening episodes which might lead to being off school sick). In these cases the accounts of both the children and their mothers suggest an active negotiating process, although as the following examples show, this process takes place within a context which shapes and constrains it.

The first example is of a child making a bid for sickness and this being resisted by his mother. Marcus described how a day off school came about:

> Well at night time I didn't feel very well and next morning I felt sick so I just stayed in bed. I told my mum but she didn't believe me at first really. But then she believed me. [AP: What changed her mind?] I don't know really, probably that I didn't get up and have my breakfast, even when she kept

calling me. [AP: Did you try and persuade her?] Sort of because when she said I should go to school I just said my stomach was hurting like.

A second situation involved a mother attempting to place a child in the sick role and meeting resistance. Kathleen, for example, hid the symptoms of her cold from her mother because she believed that she would be prevented from going swimming if it came to light. Children often seemed able to influence the timing of sickness through such tactics. Another example arose with Jenny, who was away with a 'sore throat' at the end of the spring term. She first felt ill on a Friday night but at first said nothing to her mother and a few days later, when questioned by her mother, said she felt all right. A day or so later she told her mother that her throat hurt, was examined and kept off school for a few days. Jenny explained the sequence of events:

> I wanted to do something with Miss Frazer. It was printing on Tuesday and we had to make a folder but some of them didn't turn out right so Tracy and me had to do and wanted to do it and I didn't want to be off, so on Tuesday when I felt worse and couldn't eat my breakfast properly I thought I'd better not tell my mum because I wanted to come [to school]...On Wednesday I couldn't eat anything or drink either and my eyes were all puffed up so I stayed off. My mum said to and there was nothing I wanted to do special at school.

This example begins to suggest the importance of the relationship between the temporal organization of schoolwork and sickness. The children's work in maths and English was organized according to a weekly system of 'assignments'. At the start of each week Catherine Frazer distributed a series of tasks to the children. For the rest of the week the children worked on these tasks and were expected to complete them by Friday when they were handed in for marking by Catherine. If the work was not completed the children were expected to finish it 'in their own time', usually by being kept back over playtime in the following week.

Although the children enjoyed the control over the pace of work that this system gave them, it did present them with problems if they were absent and returned to school half-way through or at the end of a week. In these circumstances they were expected to complete the assignment as usual. Just as children were active in the processes which initiated sickness, so they were able to manoeuvre around the timing of their return to school. Children's accounts frequently referred to the ways in which they attempted to align their sickness with the weekly pattern of work. An example illustrates the point. Malcolm was away from school for two weeks with tonsillitis. Towards the end of the second week his mother began to think that he was well enough to return and was worried that he had missed too long a period of schoolwork. She tried to persuade him to return to school but Malcolm insisted that he did not feel well enough. He explained to me that: 'it's the worst part of the week... mostly finishing off and that.'

It is clear then that the children, in relationship to their mothers, played an active role in the production of sickness absence, and that their negotiations were related to the temporal organization of schoolwork. This picture, however, was complicated when variations in the frequency of sickness absence over the summer term *as a whole* are taken into account. Essentially rates of absence varied in a systematic way across the period of my study and these variations were paralleled in the shifting content of the negotiations between mothers and children. In the next section I will explore the relationship of sickness to the way in which schoolwork and the time were socially organized at this level.

Work and time in the lives of 4F

The children of 4F were in the last year of English primary schooling. At the end of this particular year they would all transfer to a secondary comprehensive school and remain there until at least the age of 16. Most of the children intended to go to the local co-educational comprehensive (Lowhouse). The transition to secondary school is well documented as a major status passage in the career of English children (see for example, Measor and Woods, 1934), signifying and organizing a key moment in the extended transition from childhood to adulthood. This transition structured the form and content of the schoolwork undertaken by the children of 4F throughout their last year at Appletrees. Following Strauss et al. (1986) this work,[2] through which their transitional trajectory was constructed, is described as both instrumental and expressive related to their overall trajectory through primary schooling. The instrumental aspect flowed from the series of grading tests which the children sat during the middle of the summer term. These were in maths, English and creative writing, and were set and marked by teachers at Lowhouse school. On the basis of their performance in these tests the children were graded and placed in ability bands at Lowhouse. The tests were therefore seen by the children, teachers and parents of Appletrees as crucial to their children's future. The tests set targets which appeared as fixed and unnegotiable from the point of view of the primary school. The knowledges and skills that the tests laid down determined the schedule of the children's schoolwork, arguably throughout their time at Appletrees but certainly in a marked and urgent way through the last year. Most of this year's work centred on preparing for these tests and as they loomed nearer the more they occupied the central place in the organization of schoolwork.

The expressive aspects of this process were diffused through this period of preparation for the tests, as well as many other features of the children's lives at school. They focused on the image of secondary schooling as an altogether tougher and more competitive environment than that of primary school.[3] The aim was, to use a suggestive metaphor, making children 'fit' for the next stage of their lives. It manifested itself in many ways: the introduction of a more rigorous work discipline in the classroom; a more individualized and competitive set of work practices, such as frequent tests and mock examinations; a stress on competitive games, especially for the boys; the circulation among the children of a number of 'myths' which encoded messages about the instrumental and unemotional world they were about to enter;[4] and the increasing emphasis on the formal aspects of the curriculum, on which the children would be tested, rather than the more open-ended tasks such as project work.

In this section I will analyse the relationship between temporal aspects of the organization of schoolwork and the pattern of children's sickness during the last term. I want first to draw a theoretical distinction between what I here call 'time-work' and 'work-time', concepts which can be related to the analyses of Roth (1963) and Zerubavel (1979, 1981). According to Roth, school careers are examples found at one end of a continuum of temporal determinacy and indeterminacy: 'All participants who reach the end have passed through the same stages ... almost always in the same length of time .... There is ... no room for bargaining on the timetable' (Roth, 1963: 74).

While for Roth such apparently fixed schedules are of trivial sociological interest, for Zerubavel it is precisely their unnegotiable quality – 'rigid sequential structures, fixed durations, standard temporal locations, and uniform rates of recurrence' (1981: 1) – which stimulates the sociological imagination. For him rationalized time, 'the schedule', is a hallmark of modern societies, and not only in the familiar sense that in capitalist economic formations 'time is money'. In his celebrated study of time in hospital life, he shows how the continuous flux of time is broken into discrete segments (which he dubs 'chronemes'): the year, the rotation (of interns through various medical specialities), the week, the day and the duty period. These he suggests: 'force both routine and non-routine events and activities into regular temporal patterns, through introducing a rhythmic structure into hospital life' (Zerubavel, 1979: 35).

It is noticeable, however, that three of his rhythmic structures are, if not precise correlates, at least analogues of socially standard calendrical and clock time – the year, the week and the day. The other two, the rotation and the duty, while expressible or translatable into clock and calendrical time, are not determined by it. The temporal characteristics of the rotation and the duty period result from a particular mode of work organization, while those of the year, the week and the day impose on work organization, rhythms derived from a socially standard (but not, of course, absolute) time system. These two systems of time, which I will refer to below as respectively 'work-time' and 'time-work', interact with each other and, indeed, much of that which interests Zerubavel is a product of their intersection.

The formal organization of 4F's schoolwork was in fact represented in a timetable. It was organized according to standard clock time, necessarily so in order to ensure the internal and external coordination of the school. However, underlying and cross-cutting clock time were informal temporal rhythms associated with the organization of schoolwork. Following the terminology suggested above it is possible to distinguish these two aspects.

'*Time-work*' includes those rhythms of social life which paralleled and were based on clock and calendrical time. In Appletrees children's careers proceeded according to academic years which ran from September to September. This was divided into three terms, the length of which varied between 12 and 14 weeks. Terms were separated by holiday periods and divided into two halves by a one week 'half-term' holiday. The school week was divided into five separate days, Monday to Friday, and each day was divided into two halves defined by clock time as 9.00 am to 12.00 pm and 1.00 pm to 3.30 pm. Within each day schoolwork was organized according to a timetable which divided the day into a fixed number of work periods, usually 1 hour and 20 minutes long, interspersed by a lunch break of 1 hour and two shorter 'playtimes' of 20 minutes each. Different types of work (maths, English, etc) were fitted into the period-time units and the type of work being done changed at the end of the unit whether or not it had been completed. Standard time predominated, then, in two senses: first, it was used to coordinate the complex workings of the school, imposing on the children, for example, the duty of attending school at certain fixed times; second, it defined those periods of time in which children were expected to carry out their schoolwork, and organized them into temporal rhythms measured in socially standard units.

'*Work-time*' refers to the temporal rhythms which derived from the actual organization of schoolwork. Sometimes these coincide with time-work units so that they become difficult to disentangle from each other but nevertheless, when the organization of work is taken into account segments of time take on meaning beyond that expressed simply through their conventional subdivision of temporal flux. Seen in this light the final year and last term of primary schooling saw a concentration of work tasks and an intensificiation of the pace of work, largely in preparation for the secondary school grading tasks. In particular, the last term was not a simple equivalent of the terms that preceded it, but one in which the rhythms of work were in its first part, accelerated, and in its second, partially dissolved. The shift of these work-time rhythms turned around the secondary school tests which divided the summer term into segments which did not coincide with the formal (time-work) division of it into two half terms. The summer term was 14 weeks long and divided into two halves by a holiday in week seven. The exams took place during week four of the term. Looked at from this point of view the summer term can be divided into two halves of unequal length, separated by the exam week, and characterized by a shift in the rhythms of work.[5]

Patterns of sickness absence

Children's attendance at school was recorded in the class register which was taken by the teacher at the beginning of each morning and afternoon session. Absence was therefore counted in units of a half day and the register format provided spaces for column and row totals which the teacher was required to complete at the end of each term. Records were not kept for weekends or holiday periods. In this sense the accounting system for absence was based on time-work units which were regarded as equivalents, that is absence for one school day 'counted' as two units of absence whenever it occurred during the term or school year. This, however, was not the case in practice: absence in general, and sickness absence in particular, was regarded as less important at some times of the school year than at others and rates of sickness absence varied in systematic, work-time related ways.

I will now explore the relationship between sickness absence and the work-time rhythms which, I suggest, underlie them. The most striking feature of the work-time rhythm was the division of the summer term into two halves. The Lowhouse test took place in the penultimate week of the first half of the summer term, the halves being separated by a week's holiday. Schoolwork during the first half of the term was dominated by preparation for the tests and the content of the curriculum was modified to meet this. Throughout the fourth year most time had been devoted to maths and English, the areas of competence most directly tested by Lowhouse. In the first half of the summer term this was stepped up and 'soft' areas of the curriculum such as project work, where the children had the greatest autonomy in their learning, were reduced. Most time was given to revision and practice for the exam. For example, every Friday afternoon the children were given a 'mock' exam, using questions similar to those they would later face in the actual exam. A very formal atmosphere was created, for example

by enforcing a 'no talking' rule and forbidding any collective en-
deavour. Sickness absence at this time was particularly discouraged by
the teachers and was frequently commented upon in class.

After the tests the organization of schoolwork shifted in several
important respects: the pace became slower, there was more emphasis
on project work rather than the weekly assignments around maths and
English and more time was spent on activities such as games, swimming, drama and crafts. The tension created by the tests seemed to be
released and they were no longer dominant. In the week after the tests a
school holiday to Holland was organized and about half the children
went on it. While they were away the rest of the children also went on
day outings. The timetable was suspended, so that when, for example,
the weather suddenly turned fine, one teacher felt able to abandon
classes for the rest of the day and take the children out for a light-
hearted game of rounders.

The pattern of sickness absence was governed by these shifts in
work-time. As Table 8.1 shows sickness absence in the first half of the
term was the lowest of the year, falling outside the range of the other
half of term averages. In the last half of term, after the tests, the
sickness-absence rate increases sharply, returning to within the normal
range (and in fact slightly above the yearly average). The detail of the
week-by-week changes (shown in Table 8.2) in absence are also
revealing. The rate declined in the weeks leading up to the tests, was
very low in that week itself and rose sharply in the weeks after.

The material gathered in my study illuminates the social practices
behind this pattern, enabling a case-by-case analysis of sickness
absence. Here I have only space to illustrate the processes by which
absences occurred over this period by drawing on the following two
sets of data:

1   The contrasting parental accounts of sickness absence before and
    after the test.
2   The health diary entries before and after the test.

Table 8.1   *Average frequency of absence by half term for 4F
during academic year 1981 to 1982*

Term	Half term	Average absences per week in half days	Average absences per week over whole year
Autumn	1	16	
	2	11	
Spring	1	19	
	2	17	15
Summer	1	7	
	2	17	

By reconstructing the processes within which sickness was produced it is possible to see how work, time and sickness were related.

Parental accounts before the test

Table 8.2 shows that there were 35 sickness episodes during the whole of the summer term. Of these only 6 fell within the first part of the term defined by the test as a work-time rhythm (that is, before the tests in week 4). One of these arose after a boy was sent home ill from school in the morning. The remaining 5 involved only 3 children, one of whom was away on several occasions. I shall describe each of these cases in turn, drawing from them the features that characterize them as part of the work-time rhythm.

The first case concerns Kathleen Brindisi, who was absent for one of two days on each of the weeks immediately previous to the tests for Lowhouse entrance (Table 8.2, weeks 1, 2 and 3). The reason given by her parents on each of these occasions was the same; that Kathleen had suffered a severe nose bleed during the night or early in the morning. She had in fact a history of nose bleeds, for which she had already visited the doctor and he had arranged a hospital appointment for later in the year. When these started to recur in the summer Mr and Mrs Brindisi had been especially concerned because they were aware that this term was to be used in preparation for the Lowhouse test. Despite recognizing the importance of school performance, Kathleen's parents

Table 8.2 *Average frequency of absence and sickness absence by week for 4F in the summer term*

Week	Absences in half days	Sickness absences in half days	Number of sickness episodes	Notes
1	6	2	1	Kathleen absent
2	11	9	3	Kathleen and Sam
3	5	5	2	Kathleen and Linda
4	3	0	0	Exam week
5	n/a	n/a	n/a	School trip
6	9	8	1	
7	n/a	n/a	n/a	Half term holiday
8	12	11	5	
9	17	13	5	
10	22	2	2	
11	22	11	5	
12	21	17	4	
13	21	15	4	
14	11	9	3	

n/a = not applicable

were critical of the system, which they believed put too much pressure on children. At the same time both parents felt strongly that children must learn not to use illness as an excuse and had in the past come into conflict with Kathleen about the issue:

> All children try that on, they all go through that. She might go through another stage when she's up at Lowhouse. She might not settle and might not like it. But for the last two years we've kept having to talk to her. It's no use pretending to be ill and trying to waste time ... Sometimes I say 'Well I don't believe you, if you don't feel well you can go to school and come home again, you know I'm here.' But the chances are these days they don't.

In fact, in this case, they felt that there was no question of Kathleen feigning sickness. In the first place it did not fit into the range of symptoms which raised this suspicion for them, for example vague tummy and head aches. The symptoms were also dramatic and palpable; the nose bleeds came unpredictably and it took a long time to stem the flow. Furthermore, Kathleen had been taken to the doctor and he had confirmed that there was a physical cause to the symptoms. There still remained, however, the decision to keep Kathleen away from school. The account given to me described a trade-off which her parents had made between the costs and benefits of a sickness absence. On the one hand there were their worries about the test. On the other, Mrs Brindisi was particularly concerned about the impression she would create if she sent Kathleen to school, only to have her sent home later in the day. This was especially problematic when the symptoms, as in this case, were so messy and obvious. Mrs Brindisi therefore took a compromise track and kept Kathleen off school on the days immediately following a bad nose bleed. At the same time she took a step, unusual for her, of visiting Catherine Frazer to explain the situation and to ask that Kathleen be given work to do on those days and be excused games at school so as to reduce the risk of these causing or exacerbating the problem.

The second case is that of Sam Hunt who was away for 2 days at the beginning of week 2. Sam was a boy believed by his mother to be particularly 'soft', something she felt was evident in his tendency to complain a lot about feeling ill. On this occasion he complained about earache when he got up on Monday morning and asked if he could stay off school. Mrs Hunt felt it was important to resist such claims generally, as a way of 'toughening up' Sam in preparation for secondary school. Again she thought it especially important to insist on him going to school during this term and the tests again loomed large in her perspective. She knew that Sam was feeling anxious about the maths part of the test and felt that every day now counted if he was going to cope with it:

I know my husband has said to him that if you can't do maths you'll never get a job and not get on so he's really got to buckle down in these last few weeks. And we've been told that Lowhouse is going to be much harder. The children who've been up all say this [Appletrees] is like Butlins, so you've really got to pull the reins in.

Mrs Hunt described how she struggled with Sam about going to school that day, to the point of walking half-way to school with him and only turning back when he kept on insisting that he was really in pain:

It was the Lowhouse test and all that coming together. He said 'What'll I do if I don't pass?' but I said 'Don't be silly Sam, you're still going [to school] because you've got to learn'. [AP: Did you mean about the maths test or generally about not missing school if you feel a bit off?] Both really, because it is important he gets as much time as possible in at the moment. [AP: So what happened to change your mind?] Well it was the way he was going on on the way to school, saying how much it really hurt and that. It is very difficult when he's like that and you begin to think that there must be something in it. But I did say 'This isn't going to last too long my boy'.

The last case is that of Linda who was away for a day and a half at the end of week 3. Unlike the two previous examples, Linda's parents made no mention of the Lowhouse tests and did not seem particularly concerned about them. Their account dwelt mainly on the fact that Linda had a long-standing problem with sinusitis. I was puzzled by their lack of concern about the tests and eventually asked them how they thought Linda would do in them. At this point they told me that Linda was one of the few children in 4F not to be going to Lowhouse but to another school. This school did not stream children before entry and this led to a rather different perspective on the last term of primary school. Although they were generally concerned that Linda should not claim sickness as a way of avoiding school, they saw the last term of primary school as relatively unimportant:

I think, you know, that school life is a hell of a lot different from when I was there. The teachers seem to be a lot more easy with the pupils than they were, more opportunities, more trips, you know. I just hated school... [AP: Does she get behind if she's away?] Not a lot I don't think. She'll plod on if she's behind. I don't think Mrs Frazer thinks she's behind, not with her reading anyway. I think she's getting bored with it now and is ready to go on to her new school. I think really they've got to the stage where they can't teach them anymore 'til they get to secondary.

These cases yield insights into the process of sickness absence as it occurred in the first half of the summer term. The predominant concern was with not missing time from school which could be used in work for the Lowhouse tests. Entries into sickness were governed by their position in the work-time rhythm of the tests, as seen not only in the relatively low level of sickness but also in the character of the negotiations around the few episodes that did occur. The organization of homework for the children to do while they were absent illustrates how even during sickness time could not be taken 'off work'. At an individual level it seems that sickness occurred when the demands of work-time were offset by countervailing factors such as the patency of symptoms, the fear of being characterized as an inadequate mother or the persistence of a child's claims that they were not well. The case of Linda negatively confirms the importance of work-time as a structuring factor governing the entry of children into sickness, since the rhythms that structured sickness for most of the children did not and were not applied in her case.

Work-time is also apparent in those cases where children's claims were not transformed into sickness. In interviews with those mothers who kept health diaries through this period I was able to gather detailed accounts of how children's claims on sickness were negotiated even when they did not result in absence. During weeks 1 to 4 (from the start of the summer term to the test week) the diaries showed 24 occasions on which the children complained to their mother of feeling ill. Among this group only two such instances led to sickness absence. In 13 of the cases the mothers felt that they would not normally have kept their children away from school. In the other 11 cases it was clear that the imminence of the tests was an important feature of their negotiations and their decisions. Some examples illustrate this:

1   Nerys complained of feeling nauseous and having stomach pains but her mother felt that it was 'such an important time at school' that Nerys should not take time off.
2   André complained of hay fever. His mother went to the doctor for a preventive spray to keep it under control for the week.
3   Malcolm had sore feet in the early part of the week. His mother bathed them with salt-water every day. (The same symptoms in the next half term led to time off school.)
4   Sam complained of earache again but was sent to school. 'I was worried because it happens such a lot and I couldn't pinpoint the cause that time. But the Lowhouse test was coming up so he had to go.'
5   Rebecca complained of a cold. Her mother said that 'normally we don't take chances. We'll let her have a day off and rather be safe than sorry but it was a rather important week.'

The second half of the term

The pattern of sickness absence during this part of the term was governed by the shift in work-time which resulted from the completion of the tests. The main feature of this period was the increase in the number of sickness absences. The number of symptoms recorded by mothers in the health diaries remained approximately constant between the two halves of the term, in the second part, however, a higher proportion resulted in sickness absence. According to the health diaries there were 34 occasions on which children complained of feeling ill and 15 resulted in time being taken off school. An analysis of interviews with parents clearly shows the altered work-time situation. Again some examples can be used to illustrate this:

1 Sam was away with swollen glands and a headache for two days in June. His mother described her decision to allow him time away from school as follows:

> Anyway he came home yesterday and he did have a headache and looked white, and he didn't feel like any dinner and when they're off their food ... I said well all right, seeing as how there was nothing drastic going on down there [at school], they'll only be swimming. I knew he wouldn't miss anything terribly important and Mrs Frazer had said already that the Lowhouse tests were over anyway. So I left it like that.

2 Tina was away with a sore throat for 4 days. Her mother explained that:

> I did ask if she'd got anything she was really interested in or anything important but she said 'no, not particularly'. Obviously her maths and English, her everyday schoolwork. If she tells me there's an exam or something like that, I try and keep her at school as long as possible but of course they'd had the big one already.

3 Malcolm was away with sore feet for a day. His mother told me that:

> Nothing much seemed to be going on at school so I thought a day wouldn't do any harm now.

4 Paolo was absent with hay fever on 3 separate occasions. His mother explained that:

> I could have sent him to school but, I don't know, it didn't seem worth it by then. I feel I'm more relaxed towards it and that a day lost is never as bad as it could be. I feel that Paolo's not exactly doing badly ... Also there's that chance for me to spend an extra hour with him. It's good because we can talk together. It's as good to have a day like that as it is to send him to school. But I can be strict as well, like when they're revising.

Sickness and time economy

Thus far I have dealt with the temporal phasing of the children's last term at primary school which was produced by the social organization of their work. In particular I have focused on the 'valve' effect of the secondary school tests as it structured the uneven pattern of sickness absence by, as it were, holding back or releasing the flow of children in or out of sickness. Although I have illustrated this with examples from my fieldwork material, the patterning nevertheless tends to appear in this analysis as an external and superordinate framework imposed on the social process rather than, as I believe it was, something which grew out of the dialectic of structure and meaning within which parents, children (and teachers) acted.

In this final section then, I will further explore the relationships of time, work and sickness internal and between the two phases of the term. Each part of the term, I suggest, can be seen as constituting a contrasting economy of time (chrono-economy?), the features of which are summarized in Table 8.3.

The first part of the term was dominated by the public time of school attendance, schoolwork and the official timetable which is normative to childhood at the point of the transition to secondary school. During this phase the time scheduling of lessons was rigid, with little deviation, and the pace of children's work was firmly regulated to meet the impending and temporally fixed point of the tests. The deadline of the test meant that in this phase the economy of time was rooted in scarcity and its private consumption was subordinated to the investment of time in the public/normative work of preparation for the tests. Sickness was seen as disruptive and wasteful of time resources, which were to be saved, made and made-up. In this sense sickness stood alongside other activities such as play, games, and aspects of the curriculum seen as unnecessary to the tests; all such time expenditures were squeezed out of the economy. The children were frequently reminded of this, for example when Catherine Frazer addressed 4F about Claire's inability to cope with some of her maths:

> Now Claire, you were away a lot at the end of last term, weren't you? What was it Claire, two Wednesdays, a Monday and a Friday? And you got behind and missed the lesson where we did this. This is what can happen when you're away too often.

Table 8.3 *Contrasting economies of time in the two phases of the term*

Feature	First work-time segment	Second work-time segment
Dominant time	Public/normative	Private/individual/idiosyncratic
Time resources	Scarce	Plentiful
Time scheduling	Tight/rigid	Loose
Sickness	Saving/making	Spending/taking

The second phase of the term was a time economy of relative abundance. The tight sequencing and rigid control of lesson boundaries disintegrated, such that lessons might be switched and changed according to a variety of contingencies (for example, Graham Chapman abandoning lessons for fine weather games). At the same time the pace of work became both slower and more sensitive to the characteristics of individual children and the content shifted back to the luxuries such as games, music, drama, craft and open-ended projects previously reduced to a minimum. Into this collapse and decay of normative and public school time, percolated the consumption of time for idiosyncratic, private and individual purposes. Time that previously had had to be saved and made, became available for the taking. In this situation, sickness became aligned not only with the expansion of curriculum non-necessities ('nothing drastic going on down there') but also with the taking of in-term holidays, the fostering of individual well-being and the maintenance of personal relationships ('a chance for me to spend an extra hour with him'). Now a plentiful resource, time could be transferred for private consumption.

For 4F the transition to secondary school was a moment of extraordinary intensity, such that, as I have suggested elsewhere (Prout, 1987), it might be seen as a modified form of liminality (Turner, 1977). Unlike the 'timeless time' which Turner identifies as a feature of liminality in ritual, liminality in these children's lives appears as bifurcated systems of time, fragmenting culturally contrasting aspects of social time into specialized segments of a transition process. This sharp separation may be characteristic of periods of transition, perhaps in adulthood as well as in childhood, suggesting that such moments of social condensation deserve our special attention, allowing us to see more clearly aspects of everyday life, such as time, work and sickness, which their normally more dense entanglement renders obscure.

Notes

1. A full methodological account is given in Prout (1987). People and places have been given pseudonyms.

2. Strauss et al. (1986) argue that the term 'work' should be given a wide definition and this point coincides with the general direction of much recent sociological and anthropological theory (see, for example, Wajcman (1981) on domestic labour, Stacey (1984) on health work and Wallman (1979), Stacey (1981) and Pahl (1984) on work and the division of labour). An implication of my analysis is that schoolwork can be regarded as a form of work (alongside paid employment, domestic work etc.). On the whole the sociological importance of schoolwork has been seen in relation to social reproduction. Apple (1979: 51–60), for example, gives an excellent analysis of the work characteristics of schooling but nevertheless still identifies the sociological importance of this for the understanding of social reproduction rather than for the specific form of work central to the social construction of childhood in Western societies.

138 *Time, health and medicine*

3. See, for example, Measor and Woods (1984), which also reviews previous literature.

4. Myth here is used in the Malinowskian sense of a charter for social action.

5. In the personal and social experience of time, time-work and work-time are closely interwined in complex ways. I make the distinction for analytical purposes but in practice units of each are interconnected. For example, work periods in many English schools last 40 minutes, a seemingly arbitrary measure which may embody an historical judgement about the likely concentration span of schoolchildren. Once established, however, it is clock time which comes to define the organization of schoolwork. Teachers may try and judge the amount of work which might 'fit' into the allocated time slot available. Underlying this process, however, may be other rhythms which are generated by the work tasks themselves.

References

Apple, M.W. (1979) *Ideology and Curriculum*. London: Routledge and Kegan Paul.

Bellaby, P. (1992) 'Broken Rhythms and Unmet Deadlines: workers' and managers' time perspectives' (Chapter 7, this volume).

Gluckman, M. (1961) 'Ethnographic data in British social anthropology', *Sociological Review*, 9: 5–17.

James, A. and Prout, A. (eds) (1990) *Constructing and Reconstructing Childhood: Contemporary Issues in the Sociological Study of Childhood*. Basingstoke: Falmer Press.

Measor, L. and Woods, P. (1984) *Changing Schools*. Milton Keynes: Open University Press.

Mitchell, J.C. (1983) 'Case and situation analysis', *Sociological Review*, 31: 187–211.

Pahl, R.E. (1984) *The Division of Labour*. Oxford: Blackwell.

Prout, A. (1986) ' "Wet children" and "little actresses": going sick in primary school', *Sociology of Health and Illness*, 8(2).

Prout, A. (1987) 'An analytical ethnography of sickness absence in an English Primary School'. Unpublished PhD thesis, University of Keele.

Roth, J. (1963) *Timetables: Structuring the Passage of Time in Hospital Treatment and Other Careers*. New York: Bobbs-Merrill.

Stacey, M. (1981) 'The Division of Labour: or overcoming the two Adams', in P. Abrams et al. (eds), *Practice and Progress: British Sociology 1950–1980*. London: George Allen and Unwin.

Stacey, M. (1984) 'Who are the health workers? Patients and other unpaid workers in health care.' *Economic and Industrial Democracy*, 2(7).

Strauss, A., Fagerhaugh, S., Suscek, B. and Wiener, C. (1986) *The Social Organization of Medical Work*, Chicago: Chicago University Press.

Turner, V.W. (1977) 'Variations on a theme of liminality', in S.F. Moore and B.G. Myerhoff (eds), *Secular Ritual*. Assen: Van Gorcum.

Wajcman, J. (1981) 'Work and the Family', in *Women in Society*. London: Virago.

Wallman, S. (1979) 'Introduction' to *Social Anthropology of Work*. London: Academic Press.

Zerubavel, E. (1979) *Patterns of Time in Hospital Life: A Sociological Perspective*. Chicago: Chicago University Press.

Zerubavel, E. (1981) *Hidden Rhythms: Schedules and Calendars in Social Life*. Chicago: Chicago University Press.

9

The Dis-ease of Social Change: time and labour markets in the lives of young adults and their families

Pat Allatt

There is an accumulating body of work on the relationship between health and social change. It is underpinned by the concept of stress and its role in the onset of physical and mental illness (Rahe, 1969; Fagin and Little, 1984; Salmon, 1985). Studies range from those which consider the effect upon health of personal and expected life events, such as birth, marriage and bereavement, to investigations of the consequences of broad social change. In this latter group, particularly during the two periods of economic recession in this century, one focus has been on the effect of unemployment upon the health of individuals and their families.[1]

This chapter draws upon a study of the conjunction of personal and societal change within the family.[2] The study looked at the effect of economic recession upon the family relationships of 40 young people between the ages of 18 and 21, thus at a critical juncture in their life course, who, in the early 1980s, were living in the parental household.[3] Within this context the paper examines the impact of recession upon that sense of orderliness with which people seek to imbue their lives and which, it is argued, underpins health and well-being.

Today, definitions of health, although fraught with problems of measurement, are moving beyond a purely medical model of manifestations of physical and mental disease to take account of the well-being of the whole person (British Medical Association Board of Science and Education, 1987). This shift is reflected in the recent growth in popularity of those movements, encapsulated in the term holistic medicine, which encompass within well-being physical, mental and spiritual order. Their philosophy chimes with a concept of disease considered in this paper, embracing those underlying disjunctions and disharmonies which can be produced by social change, the uneasiness which may be the precursor of stress and malaise. Such a conceptualization of sickness is implicit in the word disease. Indeed, until the mid-seventeenth century the word had two connotations, conveying not only the modern medical meaning of disorder of the bodily organs or fluids, but also intimating uneasiness or absence of ease (*Shorter Oxford Dictionary*). While this latter interpretation may be lost to our vocabulary, that it continues to live in our culture and discourse is clear from people's descriptions of their lives and their reactions to events which disturb them.

This expanded notion of disease is explored by approaching the issue of health from the perspective of order; for the problem of order is not solely one for sociologists and social theory; it is also a problem for people in their daily lives and in their plans for the future.

Zerubavel (1981: xii, 12) elaborates the concept of order by illustrating how we regulate our lives and social world in terms of time, and Salmon (1985), discussing how people experience their lives, notes the paradox between reality, where life is constantly changing, and the sense of stability we manage to establish in our everyday lives, along with a notion of normal adult life as a time of 'settling down'.[4] In some historical periods, however, the changes associated with age, and the life events upon which we manage to impose some order and predictability, are set within the disruptive effects of wider changes. The chapter describes how the sociotemporal order we have constructed may be disrupted by events flowing from economic recession and the effect this may have upon personal well-being. There are three parts: the search for order, the disruption of order as experienced through time and the language of dis-ease.

The search for order

That people strive to impose predictability and continuity upon their lives was clear in young people's and parents' descriptions of their days and how they saw the future. This had economic, social and psychological dimensions. The many forms these took were distilled in the widespread sentiments of 'being settled', 'secure' and 'settling down', the latter, in our society, a mark of full adulthood and symbolized by marriage and actual or prospective parenthood. Consequently, given the difficulties experienced in the labour market and that the young people were on the brink of the 'settling down' process, there were many references to the interpenetrating employment and domestic careers of the lifecourse – jobs and marriage; and being 'settled in a job', meaning a 'proper' job with pay that was considered 'fair', was a recurrent theme (Allatt and Yeandle, 1986). 'Being settled', however, was also seen as a mental state, linked to security and well-being. As one mother observed: 'A person's got to be happy in their job ... I think it makes for a better world ... but if you're unsettled ....'

While 'being settled' was the goal, also conveyed was the sense that there should be an orderliness to life in general. Some responses were rooted in particular conceptualizations of time and shaped by metaphor. A perception of time as linear was associated with a view of the life course as a journey, time marked by specific events occurring at the 'proper' time in one's progression: leaving school, a job, a period of youthful enjoyment, courtship, marriage, a home of one's own and the establishment of an independent family unit or relationship. As one mother said: 'Then she started work, then she started courting, everything seemed, y'know clear'. This normative timetabling (Finch, 1987) gave way to a view of life as a flowing current along which the individual was carried, still linear but providing metaphors of interrupted flow, of eddies and backwaters. Another pattern was that of cyclical/diurnal time in the recurring schedule of the daily routine (Zerubavel, 1981). These ways of seeing and experiencing time were not mutually exclusive but intimately linked.

The dominance of the metaphor of life as a journey broadly mapped out did not mean that all followed this sequence (the route varies by social class, circumstances and education). Moreover, even in favourable times it is not without hazards; indeed, an aspect of good parenting was to put young people 'on the right foot', or 'to keep you on the right track', 'keeping the right hours and things like that'. The normative order, however, was considered proper.

This notion of ordered progression also appeared in comments on the nature and sequencing of jobs and was bound up with the idea of security – so that you could 'look forward to things', 'have prospects'. Even lowly jobs, it was felt, should contain some element of training, enabling 'you...to build up, pick things up as you go along'. Its absence accounted for the dissatisfaction young people and their parents felt about some jobs and some government training schemes.[5]

The lifelong journey and the daily routines of family life were intimately linked. Order to life was embedded in cyclical as well as linear time; for daily activities were seen as profoundly affecting the quality of the luggage you took on your journey. This view was reflected in comments on timekeeping as a mark of reliability and responsibility: children never having to be pestered to get up in the morning, parents and children being good timekeepers and not taking time off when sick. Such characteristics were the outward sign of the good worker, a reputation for which might secure you a job. In some families such traits were transmitted down the generations and shaped family routines (Allatt and Yeandle, 1986).

The underlying order and organization of the recurring days and their location in personal dispositions were revealed in the diaries respondents were asked to keep. 'Being organized' was a characteristic of this order, extending from personal tidiness to planning one's life.

'Keeping their bedroom tidy' or their personal space within it, was frequently the first response to questions about young people and household tasks. A sense of well-being or reduction in stress was associated with the pursuit of both economic and spatial orderliness. 'You've got to organize yourself when you're on the dole', said one mother where all family members were unemployed, 'because if you don't you're borrowing and ticking and worrying yourself stiff'. And a father, building an extension to the house, explained: 'Then they can all use this [working] area.... I cannot say I'm in comfort when I see washing lying around ... I cannot really relax.'

Order is a diffuse and fragile thing, intimately related to time and timing; and temporal regularity in our social world enhances our cognitive well-being (Zerubavel, 1981). Even in the best of times a sense of order is under constant construction, but unemployment, anxieties about getting or retaining a job, and the shifting or more ruthless expression of norms governing relationships between employer and employee in a labour market where labour was abundant posed greater threats to the pursuit of order and predictability. It is the impact of these wider social forces upon the temporal construction of order and the related sense of well-being to which I now turn.

The experience of dis-ease

Among the Newcastle families the disruption of temporal regularity affected life careers, the daily schedule and the participation in collective time:

> We all need to discover our sense of fit ... we need the sense of being 'on course', a trajectory on the basis of which we can anticipate, plan and hope ... a sense of meaning in life can only arise out of a reasonable expectation that plans will be fulfilled. (Parkes, 1984: 14)

Plans, however, could come to naught. For example, following the tenets of good parenting by encouraging children to pursue higher education, or even to stay on at school for an extra year, not only failed to produce the expected outcome of a good job[6] but also could leave parents with a disquieting sense of guilt: 'You feel as though you've wasted their time'. Indeed, chances of employment or training were reduced as formal age barriers were passed; even limited aspirations had to be lowered.

Moreover, seemingly ordered lives could be disrupted. Good starts became dead-ends as the labour market contracted and restructured. The effect on well-being was clear in one father's account of his own and his son's reaction to sudden redundancy. It illustrates the shattered pattern of young lives, the threats to critical staging posts in employment, domestic and consumption careers, and the underlying metaphor of sickness:

> You feel sick. I mean you say, 'Oh hell. Well what the hell is he going to do now? He's just 20 years old and where'll he get a job?' You just feel a bit sick. Plus, I mean, he's got his car now, and he's courting strong, and all of a sudden he goes from getting on and enjoying himself, buying a car, to *nothing*, and it's a big, big drop. He's been bad tempered and moody since he got finished, and that's just in a month. (emphasis in original)

It also brought to the fore latent social divisions. Some saw such progression and its consequences for health as essentially gendered, unemployment likely to affect 'the health of the lads more than it would the girls'. The rationale reflected Salmon's (1985) point, that after marriage the male journey continues to be signposted while a girl's path reaches an unmapped plateau. It was given voice in one mother's greater sympathy for the boys because 'that's been the role of a boy...that's what they function for...they leave school, they get a job, they get married, they look after a family. I mean, that's their whole purpose in life.'

Divisiveness, however, was not confined to gender; those whose expectations were so randomly crushed, especially when comparisons were made with the more fortunate, might be deflected along less legitimate pathways, posing threats to societal order as well as to parental peace of mind, but, as one mother said, 'who could blame them?'

Thus, being 'too old at 17', 'retired at eighteen' and 'back to square one' not only turned expected and anticipated journeys into unpredictable games of snakes and ladders but signified the seedbed of a more divided and unsettled society.

As well as disrupting long-term plans, economic recession penetrated the minutiae of daily life. Much has been written of how paid employment gives structure to a person's day. Engagement in the public domain of paid employment, however, impinges upon the domestic organization of the household, producing family routines and schedules. These not only provide a material order but also sustain and symbolize a moral order participation in which contributes to social solidarity. Unemployed people could find themselves marginalized from this ordering of time, living in different time worlds and unable to share in collective, time marked activities.

Time is an ambiguous and elastic entity (Wallman, 1984), and in the Newcastle study unemployment produced disorienting contrasts in the meaning and experience of time, permeating personal well-being. Those who had been in work, with tightly structured days, experiencing time as a scarce resource insufficient for their personal ends, now had time in abundance. Yet, as Jahoda et al. (1933/1972) noted, para-

doxically this expanse of time strangely contracts so that the unemployed, with more time, do less of those activities which their small
incomes can still encompass. As one father observed of his son: 'He
became . . . depressive, quiet, really quiet . . . the little things he used to
do he stopped doing . . . he basically just started to lounge around all
the time.'

There was also the contradiction between wasted time and its
importance as a strand of the still pervasive work ethic[7] where time is
seen as an irreplaceable resource, accounting perhaps for the irritation
parents felt when unemployed children spent the day idling their time
away watching television. But there was also a tension in parenting
between the imperative of the work ethic, itself underpinned by
concern for a child's future, and concern over the erosion of well-
being. One father, formerly 'a bit of a hard task master' in urging his
son to find employment, realized over the months how scarce jobs
were, becoming distressed by the changes wrought: 'I think the overall
factor was that I watched the change in him. He became morbid,
miserable, hard to communicate with, bad tempered and at the finish I
think it was hurting me more than it was hurting him.'

That unease arose from the contradictory expansion and contraction of the day, described by Jahoda et al. (1933/1972) as a return
to a more primitive and less differentiated experience of time, was
evident in attempts to impose a structure upon the hours, by for
example, engaging in activities for the unemployed, or monitoring
time and allocating activities to predetermined time slots.

As Jahoda et al. (1933/1972) also note, the situation produced
contrasting time worlds within the family. The disjunctions created
were highlighted among the Newcastle families by the issue of staying
in bed. For some, the generally accepted scheduling of time in broad
conformity with others in the pattern of sleeping and waking lost its
hold. Time patterns could be almost reversed, 'sleeping all day and
awake all night', as one mother put it, 'which causes a lot of friction'.
For others, a day starting late led to both family jibes and shock within
oneself: 'It used to be terrible, two o'clock. I used to think to myself,
"Jesus, half the day's passed away" . . . before you knew it it was
bloody tea time. She [his mother] used to say, "Oh, here he comes, the
lazy git" '.

'Staying in bed', however, was charged with deeper complexities
than upset and anger when others' sleep was disturbed. The proximity
of people who occupied different time worlds raised contradictions for
both. There was the anomaly between the morality of being up in the
morning at a 'decent' time and there being no work to go to, and the
impediments such moral conformity might cause for those who had to
meet the externally imposed deadlines of their own journeys. The

tightly scheduled business of a family getting itself off to work and school each morning was vividly revealed in the diaries; one less to account for in terms of waking, bathroom use, breakfast and 'baits' [sandwiches] eased the resources of time, space, and energy of other family members: 'I used to let them lie; one less out of the road, isn't it?'

This situation, however, created other contradictions. For those in work, the unemployed could raise the confused emotions of irritation if they were up, envy if they stayed in bed, and pity over their lack of employment. Moreover, the practices and moralities of family life could be upset. A mother's initial insistence that her unemployed sons got up at reasonable hour was undermined in two ways: first, by the illogicality of forcing them out of bed either for a futile search for work or to face an empty day, second, because their mere presence 'knocks you out of your routine', organized around domestic chores, caring for her elderly father, and her part-time job: 'It affects you more if they're in the house each day... you're sort of hanging back for them.'

Thus the symbolic order of adherence to a work ethic, witnessed in early rising, interfered with the material order of the household, posing a dilemma only resolved when her husband obtained labouring work for both boys. In Douglas's (1975) terms the unemployed, whether in bed or out of bed, were, literally, matter out of place, threatening the material and moral order.

The unemployed were out of place in other ways. Temporal symmetry denotes the synchronization of the activities of different individuals and the tendency to do many things in our lives at the same time as others, creating thereby a sense of social solidarity (Zerubavel, 1981: 65). Exclusion from collective patterns and rhythms can be stigmatizing and painful. In the Benedictine Order a common means of punishing a monk was to separate his activities temporally from the rest of the community, for example, eating meals three hours after rather than together with others. Zerubavel's (1981) example finds echoes in the experience of the unemployed as they lose their place in being part of things.

Being part of things is not confined to the activities and social relationships of work; it includes leisure, enough money to go out, appearance[8] and the numerous and seemingly trivial activities which constitute the daily round of family life. The unemployed young people had not merely lost the structure imposed by the working day but also their part in the collective flow of daily life. Not going out to work meant, ironically, they were not part of the mass deprived of time, who had to squeeze shopping into lunch hours, who were too tired to go out in the evening. They had time in abundance which had to be wasted in order to be filled: drinking coffee or lengthening the time taken to reach the job centre by taking a sister-in-law's child in a pushchair. Nor did they stand in bus queues or get crushed on public transport at peak times. They were outcasts from the solidarity arising from collective temporalities.

Temporal symmetry was disturbed in another domain. As noted, unemployed members could not easily participate in those schedules of family life prescribed by industrial time and which produce their own intimacies. A boy with 'nowt really to get up for' listened from his bed to his family's early morning routine: 'Everyone's left for work canny early, seven o'clock, eight o'clock, nine o'clock. I can hear them all talking and that.'

Nor could they participate in the family discourse of teasing and chatter. Even in caring families, unemployed members retreated physically and psychologically: 'He just lived in a world of his own . . . he just wasn't bothered with anything or anybody', said one father. 'I'm afraid she tended to go into her room quite a bit.' This mother's dilemma over her daughter staying in bed late suggests the psychologically outcast state behind such withdrawal: 'Well, I wasn't very happy about it . . . and then I just thought, "How would I have felt at her age?", and I thought, "God, I would do the same myself. I would crawl up in a blanket and hide myself".' Her daughter's lowered resistance to horseplay and teasing, leading this mother to 'speak to' her older married sons, changed dramatically when she obtained work: 'She's one of the crowd now . . . and when her brothers heard she'd started work, they were picking her up [in the air] . . . .'

The unemployed had lost access to other time-structured resources which foster belonging.[9] Living in different time worlds limited their contribution to family conversation. This was especially marked at those scheduled points in the family day, teatime for example, when members returning from the outside world of work pooled their individual experiences, 'moaned about work'; but the undifferentiated and uneventful time of those who stayed at home was already public knowledge. One boy contrasted the period on a government scheme with his present situation:

> It was like, just like being part of the . . . like closer to the family . . . like talking about things that happened . . . when they come in [now] they know that all I've been doing is sitting about . . . there's not much to talk about when I've been sitting about. I could bring up conversation when I came from work easier, much easier.

Finally, unemployment inhibited participation in temporal age-related patterns. As noted, the individual's lifecourse comprises several career strands, sometimes coinciding, sometimes conflicting (Brannen, 1987); but the sense of there being a proper time for each stage for the family/domestic career is underpinned by an expectation of its coincidence with an appropriate stage in the employment career. Unemployment throws these career timetables (Zerubavel, 1981) out of phase. 'I wouldn't encourage them to get married or anything while they're unemployed', said one mother, 'because I don't think its fair . . . to be getting married and get involved with anyone . . . I wouldn't like to think of them getting married while they were on social security and then . . . starting a family.'

It was a situation further complicated by the time-related strand of independence in that rights to independence accrue with age. The anxieties and dilemmas raised are expressed by the mother who felt that when a daughter was over 18:

> You can't say, 'Don't go out with him, and don't go out with him.' You just sort of hope that . . . they meet somebody decent, and when they do settle down it's somebody who has got . . . some qualifications maybe . . . or even a decent job. It doesn't have to be a fabulous job.

Moreover, because a normative age-related sequencing characterizes one's particular cohort, the unemployed, as they watched the courting and engagements of employed friends, could also feel excluded from the mainstream of life.

Yet the situation was set also against the knowledge that time does not stand still, that life goes on, posing the question as to whether the unemployed could or should stand aside from this flow. Several referred to being in a backwater, forgotten, thrown away. 'You just don't know when its going to end', said one mother, 'you just don't sort of see any future'.

The language of dis-ease

Work per se does not necessarily promote health; indeed some felt that their well-being was affected by deteriorating employment practices. None the less, to have paid employment was deemed important and, as illustrated above, some respondents were conscious of physical and psychological states which fluctuated with employment status. When unemployed, chronic complaints, such as psoriasis and asthma, could erupt and several reported symptoms listed in Fagin and Little's (1984) *Malaise Inventory*: moodiness, worry, irritability. Many said they had been, or were, or would very likely be, depressed, 'not that I'd hang myself, or anything like that', added one young man. It was an ambiguous, interstitial state. '[Unemployment] gets you bad tempered', said one young woman; and in phrases full of metaphor continued:

> It really wears you out. I've got a bottle there off the doctor, for depr . . . well not really depression, but just to keep going . . . but I only take it when I feel run down . . . he said I just needed a pick-me-up.

However, while people did not consider themselves to be ill, the recurrence of the word 'sick' was striking. Young people were 'sick of being on the dole', 'sick of seeing the same four walls' (after four years' unemployment), 'sick of enquiring [about jobs] and getting nowhere in a hurry', 'pig sick of being unemployed'. They noted how a boyfriend might be 'a bit sick if he didn't have a job' and how a girlfriend was 'getting sick of us going on about it'. A father recounted his reaction to his son's redundancy letter: 'he said, "I've got a letter"', and he showed it. You know, you feel *sick*' (emphasis in original).

Closely allied with expressions of sickness were those of being fed up and bored. 'I'm sick, mam, I'm fed up, I couldn't stand [unemployment]', said one girl in her search for work. The unemployed could be 'bored out of me mind' or 'not really depressed, just bored, you know, sick' – a remark from someone trying to structure his day and who felt that while unemployed greater involvement in fitness training was improving his physical health.

Lakoff and Johnson (1981) argue that the metaphors through which we interpret and shape our lives are grounded in our experience. Metaphors of sickness, boredom and being fed up have related meanings of surfeit, oppression, and disgust with overabundance, being thoroughly tired of a thing; being deeply affected by some strong feeling, producing effects similar to those of physical ailment; sickness or disorder by overfeeding (*Shorter Oxford Dictionary*). These definitions are found in the disorder and abuse of one of the body's systems.

Surfeit, oppression, disorder, and abuse in the lives of those living through recession were intimately related to their experience of time. The unemployed young people in the study suffered from several surfeits: a sense of rejection, of low income and also of time. Not only had they too much, but time itself was disordered, affecting them and intruding upon other. They were out of phase with those rhythms and flows of life which our society considers normal. They felt abused, unfairly treated by the wider society.

The endemic issue of staying in bed can be viewed from this perspective. The tensions and paradoxes created have been noted; the rationales included laziness, being in the way, no point in getting up. Yet to stay in bed is part of the sick role. Sick people stay in bed.[10] Here, however, it produced a mixture of censure, sympathy, and an awareness that it could actually be bad for you, 'lead to bad habits' for life and a continued disjunction with the rest of the world. It could be, however, that retreat to bed was not mere overindulgence but a sign of the underlying disorder and dis-ease into which the unemployed were thrust. The mother's empathy with her daughter, noted earlier, carried this connotation; wounded animals would crawl away and hide, either to aid recovery or to die.

The metaphor of sickness also appeared in instances which not only suggested the adoption of the sick role but also a latent hierarchy in the relationships between employed and unemployed. Visits to the unemployed were described in the idiom of sick-visiting: 'there was two girls who work where I'm working now, and they really, they were really good. They kept coming and seeing us and all that.'

Fagin and Little (1984) argue that, because unstigmatized, the sick role is easier to bear than that of unemployment. The sick role, however, has other dimensions. It was not that the girl was ill but rather that adoption of the passivity, gratefulness and subordination contained in the comment, and which characterize the good patient, possibly helped the relationship with employed friends.

Metaphors which structure our thought and action form coherent systems across physical, cultural and intellectual domains of concepts (Lakoff and Johnson, 1981). The metaphors of sickness were embedded in a text replete with words and phrases depicting subordination of the individual, both of the inner self and in relationships with others. Several appear in the earlier quotations, a few examples of such phrases will suffice here: 'down in the dumps', 'gets you down', 'pulls you down', 'gets you down inside', 'pulls your confidence down', 'sets me back', '[employed friends] feel above you, they suddenly change', 'degrading at this age, the feeling that nobody wants you', 'stripped of their dignity', 'it's sad', 'just like idling away', 'stuck on the dole', 'on the scrapheap', 'broke her heart'.

These reflect elements of Lakoff and Johnson's (1981) system of 'UP–DOWN' spatialization metaphors. They note that: 'General well-being: happiness, health, life, control and status, has the general orientation of being up . . . Serious illness forces us physically to lie down. When you are ill you are physically down' (Lakoff and Johnson, 1981: 297). It was these elements of well-being that were threatened by the dis-ease produced by disordered time. The grounds of incipient sickness were there and surfaced in the idiom through which people described their experiences.

Conclusion

This chapter draws attention to the disorientations and disjunctions in time experienced by young people still living in their parents' households. The data are drawn from a small group of 40 families living in the north-east of England and it is therefore unwise to generalize the findings, although similar disruptive effects have been noted by other researchers. Among the Newcastle families this disturbance to the ordering of people's lives, flowing from societal change beyond their control, ranged from the interruption and disruption of culturally

defined life plans and expectations to the participation in the daily
rhythms of collective life, especially as it was experienced within the
family. Such disorder, it is argued, creates a profound sense of dis-ease
for the individual, both personally and in relationships with parents
and siblings as well as with acquaintances outside the family.

Two hundred years ago such disordered states formed one definition
of disease. The data suggest that, although not retained in medical
terminology and practice, such a definition has continued to live in our
idiom and culture. People in the study described their reactions to
unemployment in terms of sickness set within a vocabulary of subordination. Together they constituted a cohesive system of metaphor
which indicated a lack of well-being. This is not to say that to be
unemployed is to be sick. Experience of unemployment varies, and for
some health may improve. However, if unemployment and even job
uncertainty is experienced as the state of dis-ease as described in this
chapter, then this could provide the underlying conditions conducive to
the malaise and physical and mental disorders revealed in other
studies. It is a salutary thought that today's economy renders so many
vulnerable to such dislocation.

Notes

1. The connections between unemployment, the ensuing drop in income and ill
health are open to debate. Carr-Hill (1987) argues that the claim that unemployment *per
se* affects physical health is rarely evidenced. Platt (1986: 151), however, notes studies
which he claims 'point unequivocally to a deterioration in physical health caused by
unemployment'.
2. The study, funded by the Leverhulme Trust, and now reported in Allatt and
Yeandle (1992), was of the effect of unemployment on 40 young people (approximately
half males and half females aged between 18 and 21 years of age) and their families, living
in a working class neighbourhood of Newcastle upon Tyne, locally acknowledged as
having a strong work ethic. Most of the young adults had experienced unemployment,
but at the time of interview, 1983 and 1984, approximately half were in paid work,
although this might be part-time or temporary. Most of the young people had left school
at 16 with few qualifications, some had stayed on for a year. One older brother was a
graduate and unemployed. Most were living with their parents: one girl had left because
of the tensions created by her unemployment and was living with her married sister; one
boy, brought up in a local authority home, was sharing a flat with a friend. Families with
sick members were excluded as it was felt that problems associated with sickness would
override unemployment effects.
3. Analysis of 1980 census data suggests that most young people in our society
remain in the parental home until they either leave to marry or cohabit. In 1980, 43 per
cent of women and 63 per cent of men were still doing so at the age of 21 (Kiernan, 1985).
4. In everyday speech the term 'settle' denotes the establishment of calm, a return to
a state of equilibrium or comfort: we settle our debts, our differences and our stomachs,
we settle in, settle down and settle up.
5. The Manpower Services Commission (later the Training Agency) established and

funded by central government, operated a range of training schemes (since 30 April 1990 contracted to the Training and Enterprise Councils) for school leavers and young people. Many of the young people interviewed had participated in the Youth Opportunities Programme (YOP) in which placements were normally of six months' duration. This was superseded by the Youth Training Scheme (YTS), at first (1983 to 1985) offering twelve-month placements and extended in April 1986 to a two-year programme for 16 year olds and one year for 17 year old school leavers.

  6. The character of local labour markets may be more important to a young person's job prospects than qualifications and social background (Ashton and Magquire, n.d.).

  7. There is little evidence of a decline in the significance most people attach to paid work, and elements of the work ethic show a continuing resiliance. This is not to suggest that large sections of the population hold a precise understanding of the behaviour patterns and values which Weber propounded as components of the ethic – asceticism, hard work, the morality of work itself, that time is money – rather people have a 'feel' of the ethic (Brock, 1985).

  8. One mother commented: '[It] makes them feel *more* out of it. They're out of it as it is when they can't get work, without being out of fashion as well.'

  9. Contrasting time worlds and their consequences are also found among those in paid work. A father on night work explained that his ignorance of family events and decisions was not due to his lack of interest but to his work schedule.

  10. I would like to thank Ronald Frankenberg for drawing my attention to this.

References

Allatt, P. (1986) 'The Young Unemployed: Independence and Identity', in B. Pashley (ed.), *Youth Unemployment and the Transition to Adulthood*, Papers in Social Policy and Professional Studies, 4. Hull: Department of Social Policy and Professional Studies, University of Hull.

Allatt, P. and Yeandle, S.M. (1986) 'It's Not Fair Is It?: Youth Unemployment, Family Relations and the Social Contract', in S. Allen, A. Watson, K. Purcell and S. Woods (eds), *The Experience of Unemployment*. London: Macmillan.

Allatt, P. and Yeandle, S.M. (1992) *Youth Unemployment and the Family: Voices of Disordered Times*. London: Routledge.

Ashton, D. and Maguire, M.J. (n.d.) *Young Adults in the Labour Market*, Department of Employment Research Paper 55. London: Department of Employment.

Brannen, J. (1987) 'The Resumption of Employment After Childbirth: a Turning Point Within a Life Course Perspective', in P. Allatt, T. Keil, A. Bryman and B. Bytheway (eds), *Women and the Life Cycle: Transitions and Turning Points*. London: Macmillan.

British Medical Association Board of Science and Education (1987) *Deprivation and Ill Health*. London: British Medical Association.

Brock, P. (1985) 'Why the Unemployed Are Getting the Blame Being Jobless', *The Guardian*, 1 May.

Carr-Hill, R. (1987) 'The Inequalities in Health Debate: a Critical Review of the Issues', *Journal of Social Policy*, 16(4): 509–53.

Douglas, M. (1975) *Implicit Meanings: Essays in Anthropology*. London: Routledge and Kegan Paul.

Fagin, L. and Little, M. (1984). *The Forsaken Families*, Harmondsworth: Penguin.

Finch, J. (1987) 'Family Obligations and the Life Course', in A. Bryman, B. Bytheway, P. Allatt and T. Keil (eds), *Rethinking the Life Course*. London: Macmillan.

Jahoda, M., Lazarsfeld, P.F. and Zeisal, H. (1933/1972) *Marienthal*. London: Tavistock.

Kiernan, K.E. (1985) 'Leaving Home: a Comparative Analysis of Six Western European Countries', Paper Presented at ESRC Workshop 5: *Problems of Methodology in Family and Household Research*. Manchester.

Lakoff, G. and Johnson, M. (1981) 'Conceptual Metaphor in Everyday Language', in M. Johnson (ed.), *Philosophical Perspectives on Metaphor*. Minneapolis: University of Minneapolis Press.

Parkes, C.M. (1984) 'Foreword' in L. Fagin and M. Little, *The Forsaken Families*. Harmondsworth: Penguin Books.

Platt, S. (1986) 'Recent Trends in Parasuicide ("attempted suicide") and Unemployment Amongst Men in Edinburgh', in S. Allen, A. Watson, K. Purcell and S. Woods (eds), *The Experience of Unemployment*. London: Macmillan.

Rahe, R.H. (1969) 'Life Crisis and Health Change', in May and Winterborn (eds), *Psychotropic Drug Response: Prediction Studies*. London: Thomas.

Salmon, P. (1985) *Living in Time*. London: Dent.

Wallman, S. (1984) *Eight London Households*. London: Tavistock.

Zerubavel, E. (1981) *Hidden Rhythms. Schedules and Calenders in Social Life*. Berkeley: University of California Press.

10

Time and Health Implicated: a conceptual critique

Barbara Adam

Time and health are the central themes of this volume. As focus of attention they have generated a wealth of information and ideas. Yet, as phenomena and in their relation they have remained strangely elusive. They have retained a quality of invisibility despite being the focus of the investigations. The studies demonstrate that time is implicated in every aspect of social being: time has occurred in association with deadlines and waiting, with negotiation of absence and work rhythms, and with the production schedules of an industrial and a medical kind. In doctor–patient interactions it has emerged in relation to efficiency and empathy, to a patient's or a disease's history, and to consultants' measurable commitment to their work. Time has further been utilized as finitude – the ontological condition of life unto death – as a resource to be used, allocated or controlled, as a commodity to be exchanged for money, and as a symbol expressive of the unequal distribution of power. Lastly, time issued as duality of structure, constructing social life and constructed by it, and as a parameter within which to achieve, fail and fall victim to stress. Despite this complexity of conceptualizations, however, time has largely remained an implicit, untheorized category of the studies. A social science focus on the time aspects of health, it seems, does not necessarily bring these into high relief or explore their relation. It does not break through their taken-for-granted status. It assumes that we know what is meant. As quantity, quality, rhythm, chronology, history and intensity the time aspects of health form unproblematic components of the analyses.

Health too has remained mysteriously invisible, despite the analytical distinctions of illth, illness, disease and sickness. Here the conceptualization of illth has been suggested as the appropriate opposite to health, illness as the pre-patient definition of illth from the perspective of the unwell person, and disease as the abstracted diagnosis of the patient's ailment by the biomedical professional. Lastly, sickness has been proposed as a conceptualization that can highlight the social nature of health. As socially constructed and constructing sickness has been argued to be maintained and recreated in an ongoing contextual social process. Yet, despite these reconceptualizations, health is still curiously intangible.

The relation between time and health is conceptualized in a variety of ways. For Bellaby (Chapter 7) it entails the timing of sickness within a context of social schedules as well as the sources of sickness in terms of broken rhythms and unmet deadlines. Prout (Chapter 8) proposes conceptualizations of 'work-time' and 'time-work' to demonstrate the mutual structuring of clock and calendar time on the one hand, and the time arising from the context dependent, negotiated pattern of sickness absence on the other, while Pritchard (Chapter 5) stresses the inappropriately one-sided response of general practitioners to their patients and argues the need for 'time empathy'.

In some of the studies the social nature of time and health is asserted or assumed from the outset. This excludes as irrelevant the times of our body and the natural environment and it avoids an involvement with ontological issues. This approach has a long tradition in social science and is based on two underlying beliefs: that science has no base from which to study the nature of phenomena and that the times of nature lie outside the boundaries of social science enquiry. Existential issues and questions of ontology, it is reasoned, belong to the realm of philosophy and metaphysics and natural time to biology and physics. Recognizing the tradition and accepting the difficulty I nevertheless want to suggest that this position is in need of reassessment. Luhmann pin-points the dilemma well when he writes:

> Normally neither historians nor sociologists ask about the nature of time. If this question is posed directly and framed as one about essences, it cannot be adequately answered. On the other hand, there is a substantial danger that, if we leave this question unaddressed, we shall think about social history in crude and inadequate ways. (Luhmann, 1982: 299)

For Luhmann this applies not only to social history but to the social sciences. For him *the philosophical theory of time is a necessary precondition for an adequate social theory*. Temporality, he insists, is a constitutive dimension of the subject matter of social science which means that 'time can no longer be treated merely as a category underlying our knowledge of social life' (1982: 290). Work which demonstrates that necessity has recently been undertaken (Bergmann, 1981; Adam, 1990). It shows first that questions of the origin, source and nature of phenomena are regularly converted into questions of meaning, and second how this simple translation reabsorbs phenomena into the sphere of the taken-for-granted. The exclusion of the times of nature from social science analysis has also been shown to be highly problematic and in urgent need of reassessment (Adam, 1988, 1990; Young, 1988). I want to propose here that natural time is integral to social time and that we have to begin to understand the multiple times of existence in relation to each other. Furthermore, I intend to show that an *explicit* focus on both time and health not only lifts their respective cloaks of invisibility but leads to insights on the relation of time and health which in turn have significant implications for our understanding of social life.

In this chapter I therefore want to sketch a picture of the mutual implication of time and health and highlight the conceptual changes arising from it. I want to look at the relation of time and health as it arises from contemporary scientific studies, from medicine, psychiatry and psychotherapy and to explore the effects of such an understanding for both theory and practice.

The times of nature and the body are inseparable from human being, from well-being and from everyday social life. The studies collated by Luce (1973) in her book *Body Time* demonstrate how rhythmicity, temporality and tempo are fundamental to our being and how their particular interplay signifies health, ill health or even death.

As living beings we are permeated by rhythmic movements which range from very fast chemical and neuron oscillations, by way of slower waves of heartbeat and respiration, to menstrual and reproductive cycles, and to the very long-range ones of climatic changes. What is important to appreciate, as Fraser (1982: 145) points out, is that 'the cyclic behaviour of all organisms involves the collective, orchestrated temporal programs of all these processes together'. Activity and rest alternations, cyclical exchanges and transformations, seasonal and diurnal sensitivity, all form the silent pulse of our being. They seem to constitute those aspects of life we take most for granted:

> Though we can neither see nor feel them, we are nevertheless surrounded by rhythms of gravity, electromagnetic fields, light waves, air pressure, and sound. Each day, as the earth turns on its axis, we experience the alternation of light and darkness. The moon's revolution also pulls our atmosphere into a cycle of change. Night follows day. Seasons change. The tides ebb and flow. And these are echoed both in animals and in man. (Luce, 1973: 16)

Not just everything we do, but all of our body's physiological processes are *temporally organized and orchestrated*. We eat, sleep, breathe, use energy, digest, perceive, think, concentrate, communicate, interact and work in a rhythmic way. All the processes of our body are accurately timed and paced so that our organs, tissues and hormones are produced at mutually related rates. The food we eat would poison us were it not for a surge of activity of kidney and liver enzymes which, in turn, had to be produced ready for accelerated action.

Daylight and darkness act as cues to keep us synchronized with our environment and this circadian cycle (circadian = circa one day) is an important organizing principle of our physiology. Desynchronization, on the other hand, express itself through loss of health (Aschoff, 1965, 1981, 1983; Brown et al., 1970; Conroy and Mills, 1971; Cloudsley-Thompson, 1980; Fraser, 1987; Young, 1988; Rose, 1989). Our body temperature, blood pressure, respiration, and pulse, our haemoglobin and amino acid levels, our hormone production, and our liver, urine and kidney function, our cell division, even our strengths and weaknesses rise and fall within this circadian cycle (Luce, 1973: 112–36; Aschoff, 1983; Rose, 1989). Within this circadian variation each of the processes takes a different 'length of time' to complete one cycle. We breathe, for example, 15 to 20 times per minute while our heart beats 60 to 80 times during the same period. While we are awake we show observable cycles of activity and rest of about 90 to 100 minutes. These may vary with age, body size, and between individuals. Our digestive system takes on average three hours to complete a cycle before we begin to be hungry again.

Day and night are not the only environmental rhythms to which we respond. This is demonstrated by menstrual cycles, seasonal growth, and the cyclical variation in hormone levels and certain illnesses (Luce, 1973: 217–31). Even the occurrences of birth and death shows seasonal variation. Through such common ideas as winter gloom and spring fever, winter cold, hay fever, and summer flu we acknowledge the influence of seasons on our health. Thus, our multiple body rhythms are not only orchestrated into a coherent whole but are also synchronized with the rhythms of the environment. This applies to all living organisms.

Sunlight as radiant energy seems to be one of the most important forces which tunes us, along with most other living creatures, to the cycles of our earth. In contradistinction to other creatures, however, we are influenced by another light source: our created artificial light. With this technological aid we have begun to 'colonise the night' to use Melbin's (1987) phrase. Those hundred years of being able to light the natural hours of darkness have to be seen in relation to our circadian evolutionary history. While humans are the most flexible beings in terms of the range within which they can vary their body rhythms, electricity has not existed for long enough to make physiological adaptive changes, as Aschoff's experiments in lightproof conditions show (1965, 1981, 1983). Our body rhythms have evolved in conjunction with the dark–light cycle of our earth and there is a limit to the adaptive changes of which we are capable within this miniscule time span of evolution. Inverting day and night, crossing time zones, keeping long, erratic hours and working rotating shifts all predispose us to desynchronization of these finely tuned and orchestrated rhythms (Luce, 1973; Rinderspacher, 1985; Young, 1988; Rose, 1989).

Sociologists make much of the modern dominance of clock time and its effect on our social lives and institutions, neglecting that we also *are* clocks that resonate with the multiple pulses of our earth and that bind us to nature's rhythms. The rhythms of our body and of the natural environment need to be recognized in conjunction with our socially constructed clock time and with technological achievements such as electricity and aviation. The last have fundamentally altered our sleep–rest patterns. In extreme cases they have stressed our capacity to synchronize and calibrate our multitude of physiological and social rhythms. Lack of concentration, tiredness and fatigue, even accidents and illness may be the outcome as research on shift work and aviation shows (Reinberg and Ghata, 1965; Dirken, 1966; Reinberg et al., 1984; Folkard and Monk, 1985; Rinderspacher, 1985). Social life organized around the clock has shifted the emphasis of everyday living and working patterns *from variable rhythms to invariant ones*. This tension is clearly demonstrated in the papers by Pizzini and Bellaby (see Chapters 4 and 7) and in the studies of Thompson (1967), Clark (1982), Rinderspacher (1985) and Young (1988). The invariability of clock-time rhythms, sudden changes in established rhythms, and the superimposition of rhythms, they all affect our well-being.

So far I have predominantly focused on natural rhythms not because I think them more important but in order to redress a traditional social science imbalance and to enable me to show those multiple rhythms in relation to each other. It is principally important not to lose sight of the many general multiple rhythms during the study of the particular. The explicit focus on any one, I suggest, must fundamentally implicate all others.

Contained within the rhythmic organization of our body are speed, sequencing, timing, prioritizing, and spacing of single actions and cycles. These structural aspects of rhythmicity apply equally to the rhythms of the body and to those of social life. In the normal course of daily life we time, sequence, prioritize and pace our activities without much conscious thought and the organization of our body rhythms certainly does not need our conscious attention. Getting up, having breakfast, catching the bus, doing homework or a balance sheet, cooking dinner and reading a patient's history all get done knowing first how long these activities take, and secondly when and how fast they need to be done in relation to other activities, other demands, and available time. A sense of urgency arises, and with it *enforced conscious decision-making*, when we encounter either a sudden shift in the routine of established rhythms, or when more needs to be done than appears possible within the available session, day, month, or years. Again the structural similarities of the time aspects of the body to those of everyday activities are striking. Both are stress-producing situations and time is the common denominator that allows us to synthesize what are otherwise isolated symptoms. Orchestrated cycles of activities when desynchronized or speeded up may best be conceptualized as stress which in turn may result in ill health and accidents. The conceptual cluster of rhythmicity, desynchronization and stress allows us to see both the structural relatedness and the inseparability of physical, physiological and social processes. Fused these processes constitute the difference between well-being and ill health.

Not just physiological well-being but mental health too is associated with the rhythms of our body. Without being able to establish causal connections or understand the relations, it has been noted that problems of mental health and desynchronization correlate (Luce, 1973: 103–5; Payk, 1979: 86, 118; Heimann, 1983: 75). Mental health is, however, not only identifiable by the harmonious orchestration of the rhythms of our biological and social being but also with reference to how we orientate in time and how we relate to the times of the world around us, our identity, and the past, present and future (Merloo, 1970; Estrote, 1982; Melges, 1982).

Orientation in, relation to, and the usage of time can act as indicators of mental health. To be considered a sane adult person in our society requires that we are able to locate ourselves along the continuum of past, present and future: our own and our societies' history and projected future. To be our own past, to have a past, and to be able to look back on it, contemplate it, and reconstruct it in terms of present values, goals and perspective, all this should form an unproblematic, seamless unity. It should present no problem. We are also expected to be able to locate ourselves in the public time of calendars and clocks and the natural time of days, nights and seasons. We are supposed to know their sequence, duration and characteristics. Binding past and future, as well as public and private time into our active present should be something we do continuously and without conscious effort. When these taken-for-granted time actions become a problem of daily living we begin to recognize once more the mutual implication of time and health.

Persons suffering from Korsakow Syndrome bring into sharp relief what is normally assumed as natural and therefore invisible: what it means to be able to orientate in time and to have a time perspective. Such persons have no means of differentiating between events that have happened very recently and those which lie in the long distant past, nor can they distance their present from their past. They are neither able to live as historical beings nor capable to locate themselves biographically in an objective grid of time. This entails that they are no longer able to respond to present situations or plan the future. Scheller (1963: 83) argues that the problem of persons suffering from Korsakow

Syndrome is not to be interpreted as merely a loss of the ability to memorize and order events, or to locate them in public time, but more fundamentally as an *inability to recognize and reflect one's own becoming.* Sufferers cannot locate their own changing being with reference to the past and future. The moment is experienced as a now only. It lacks the extension of a present that fundamentally implies past and future. Not merely a problem of memory, as originally defined by Korsakow at the turn of the century (Payk, 1979: 64), the Korsakow Syndrome signifies an incapacity to reflect one's becoming and an inability to orientate within birth–death and social history. This turns life into an insoluble dilemma for the afflicted.

To locate the self as actor within a seamless unity of past, present and future, social history, and objective time is something we take for granted until this capacity breaks down. Only then do we begin to recognize its nature through the devastating effects. The lack of this capacity, which also applies to persons suffering from schizophrenia, deprives those afflicted of a feeling of continuity, a sense of self, and a reality-constructing time perspective. Schizophrenia sufferers complain further of a splitting up of time into a multitude of separate parallel bits of time, which is accompanied by a breakdown of cohesion and order of past, present and future. For some patients space-time and even the self are experienced as dissolving into nothingness. The past and future become interchangeable, and superimposed upon each other they leave no room for a reality constructing present (Bister, 1963; Estrote, 1982; Payk, 1979; Heimann, 1983). The capacity to locate ourselves and to orientate in time thus constitutes tacit criteria for sanity. Confronted with its breakdown we become able to see the invisible.

This also applies to our relationship to time. Living predominantly in the past or the future, the characteristics of depression and mania respectively, is generally recognized as contrary to a healthy relation. When old people not merely reminisce but begin to live their present in the past we draw the line between what most healthy elderly people tend to do and illness. Through it we can recognize the healthy relation to time as one where the present is constructed within a horizon of past and future and where the latter are meaningfully integrated and constituted.

Rhythmicity, periodicity, appropriate tempo, sequencing, and timing, however, do not disappear simply because we have focused on issues of orientation in and relation to time. Not only are our own and our society's rhythms and times maintained but the illness itself is constituted by its own superimposed temporality, rhythmicity, tempo, and past, present and future. Rhythms within rhythms within rhythms, orchestrated and synchronized, and located within the birth–death parameter can vary in intensity, coordination and timing. The demarcation between health and non-health is a fluid and relative one.

The picture is further complicated by an entire area not focused on in this essay: growth and ageing. As the processes where decay and regeneration stand in a particular relation to each other, growth and ageing are inextricably bound to birth and death which in turn permeate our existence. Together they constitute our temporality and are not separable from the other times of our being. The tempo of an action, for example, is not only relative to the metabolism and temperature of beings and their observers but it also varies with age and the habits, past experiences, likes and dislikes of individuals. We know that time passes much slower for young children than for the elderly. A birthday tomorrow can seem like an eternity to a three year old while older persons tend to experience the years between birthdays flying past as if they were days. Yet, irrespective of age, we can all lose track of time when we are deeply engrossed in an activity while minutes can seem like hours when we are in pain.

Looking at the time aspects of health thus illuminates not merely their mutual implication but gives us some indication of the nature of health and time. An explicit focus on time affords insights on health while looking at non-health helps to make visible what we take most for granted: the complex times of our being. What emerges as important, however, is not only the interpenetration of time and health but the mutual implication of all the aspects of time we have focused on. In other words, all expressions of rhythmicity, periodicity, temporality, tempo, timing, orientation in time, and relation to time have to be appreciated *together* if we want to get a sense of the connections between time and health.

So far I have stressed the structural continuity of the time base of physiological, socio-mental and social processes. There is, however, one discontinuity which is of deep significance for our well-being: clock time. It fundamentally differentiates the rhythms of nature from social rhythms.

Clock time, the organizational time frame and structure of industrial production, is governed by the non-temporal principle of invariant repetition. Objectified and reified it is related to as a quantity. Social rhythms structured by the clock are thus fundamentally different from the rhythms of nature which entail repetition with variation, the essence of temporality. *What constitutes life for one spells failure for the other.* Abstracted from its natural source machine time is created to the goal of invariability and perfect predictability. As such it becomes an absolute: an abstract value to be exchanged and bought on the labour market, a finite quantity to be used, allocated, budgeted and controlled.

Both types of rhythms constitute parameters because it is repetition that facilitates prediction, foresight and planning. However, while natural rhythms fundamentally entail becoming, the created cycles of clock time, severed and abstracted from the natural source, have become a measurable, finite quantity. Not only are our bureaucratically organized, clock-time based rhythms at odds with our natural ones but they have become so pervasive that we think of them as being time per se. Conceptualizing our created, invariable time as *being* time affects our understanding of reality and our assumptions about human beings and their societies. This losing sight of temporal time, and viewing as an unproblematic unity what is distinct and fundamentally different, affects the way we relate to time as social beings, as healers and as social scientists.

Only the quantity of machine time, I propose, is limited. It is finite because it excludes becoming. It does not create time in the present but it *is* time: a time that is running on and out. This finite resource, this quantity which is running out, is a phenomenon that belongs *exclusively* to societies that have created time and relate to their creation as being time per se. As such clock time forms an integral part of contemporary Western societies' time consciousness. It thus needs to be recognized in its distinctiveness and has to be accounted for as such in contemporary social analyses. However, while social scientists are almost entirely concerned with the measurable quantity, Bergson (1888), (1932), and leading contemporary physicists such as Bohm (1980) and Prigogine (1980) have theorized time predominantly with reference to its natural temporality. I want to suggest that we have to understand the time of the clock *together with* the temporality of processes, things, people and their interactions since contemporary Western social existence fundamentally entails both. We have to begin to see them together and as inseparably linked. To study in relation what has thus far been treated as isolated domains of scientific enquiry can shift our view of the mutual implication of time and health to a new level of understanding. I have demonstrated elsewhere the cohesion and the unity of conception and assumptions of Newtonian physics, Cartesian philosophy and created machine time (Adam, 1988, 1990). In this chapter I want to begin to relate these findings to our assumptions about health.

We see ourselves as individuals and assume our bodies to be material objects, occupying space and existing for a finite time. Like atoms, which we believe make up the ultimate building blocks of our body, we see ourselves moving in space which takes time. Matter, space and time are assumed absolute. Neither creatable nor destructible, space, time, and matter *are*. The behaviour of matter, we think, is governed by causal laws, locatable in space and measurable by time. This view of space, time and matter is no longer supported by the findings and understandings of leading contemporary physicists who have established temporality as fundamental, and temporal time as a law of nature. A time that constitutes the present and principally includes becoming and repetition with variation is neither finite nor useable as a quantitative measure. Time running out, I want to propose, is a conceptualization which is exclusive to a clock-time understanding of the world. As such it is at variance with temporal time. Time efficiency, time budgeting, time management, they all belong to the clock-time conceptualization of time.

But what of health? What is the significance of that difference with respect to our well-being? Dossey (1982) writes of 'hurry sickness'. He associates a great number of diseases with the speeded-up pace of living, the pressure of getting things done in time, and the pervasive feeling of time running out. I want to propose that these kinds of time-based diseases are premised on a clock-time concept of finite time: a time that is a quanitifiable, measurable, usable resource and a parameter for achievement. Deadlines, time management and the ever-increasing pace of life, I suggest, have to be understood in relation to clock time. They are meaningless with respect to the embedded, creative and constitutive times of nature. Yet they do affect our physiological well-being. Dossey (1982) shows how an intense sense of urgency speeds up our body rhythms with the frequent outcome of heart disease, high blood pressure, a lowering of the immune function and an increase in susceptibility to infection and cancer:

> Having convinced ourselves through the aid of clocks, watches, beeps, ticks, and a myriad of other cultural props that linear time is escaping, we generate maladies in our bodies that assure us of the same thing – for the ensuing heart disease, ulcers, and high blood pressure reinforce the message of the clock: *we* are running down, eventually to be swept away in the linear current of the river of time. For us, our perceptions have become our reality. (Dossey, 1982: 50)

The more severe the illness, the more the message that time is running out becomes pertinent since it enforces a confrontation with death and finality. Many have noted fear as the dominant contemporary response to death and have interpreted much of our social endeavours and our health care as a response to that fear (Mitford, 1963; Becker, 1973; Aries, 1976). Fear, however, elicits physiological responses very similar to those already encountered in stress states where hurrying after unmet deadlines within ever diminishing finite time is associated with increased heart rate and high blood pressure. We can now see the cycle closing to an invariant circle going round and round: a finite quantity of time which is running down and out, stress, disease, fear of death, time running out, stress, disease fear of death *ad infinitum*.

Medical practitioners and other healers have found that time-slowing strategies such as meditation, biofeedback, imagery, hypnosis, and autogenic training can be used to intercept that closed circle and to counteract those contemporary time diseases (Dossey, 1982; Graham, 1990: 108–85). If, however, we want to effect changes that pre-empt the diseases rather than attempt a cure, then I suggest, it becomes essential that we bring time in its multiple expressions to the conscious level of our understanding. We need to begin to recognize the difference and the continuity between the times of becoming and the time of created invariability, the times of life and the time of death. We need to lift time from the level of the taken-for-granted meaning to an understanding that knows the relation between the finite resource, birth–death and being–becoming, between chronology, the seasons and growth. We need to de-alienate time: reconnect clock-time to its sources and recognize its created machine character. Temporal time, the symbol of life, needs to be allowed to take a position of high visibility. Recognizing time running out as our creation, temporal time as present-creating becoming, and both as fundamental to our social life gives us not only choice but it enables us to re-view the mutual implication of time and health.

References

Adam, B.E. (1988) 'Social Versus Natural Time, a Traditional Distinction Re-examined', in M. Young and T. Schuller (eds), *The Rhythms of Society*. London: Routledge. pp. 198–226.

Adam, B.E. (1990) *Time and Social Theory*. Cambridge: Polity Press. Philadelphia: Temple V.P.

Aries, P. (1976) *Western Attitudes toward Death. From the Middle Ages to the Present*, translated by P.M. Ranum. London: Marion Boyars.

Aschoff, J. (ed.) (1965) *Circadian Clocks*. Amsterdam: North Holland.

Aschoff, J. (ed.) (1981) 'Biological Rhythms', *Handbook of Behavioural Neurobiology*, vol. IV. New York: Plenum Press.

Aschoff, J. (1983) 'Die innere Uhr des Menschen', in A. Peisl and A. Mohler (eds), *Die Zeit*. München: Oldenburg Verlag. pp. 133–44.

Becker, E. (1973) *The Denial of Death*. New York: The Free Press, Macmillan.

Bergmann, W. (1981) *Die Zeitstrukturen Sozialer Systeme: Eine Systemtheoretische Analyse*. Berlin: Duncker and Humblot.

Bergson, H. (1888/1910) *Time and Free Will*. London: Swan Sonnenschein.

Bister, W. (1963) 'Über die Zeiterfahrung des Schizophrenen', in G. Schaltenbrand (ed.), *Zeit in nervenärztlicher Sicht*. Stuttgart: Ferdinand Enke. pp. 49–54.

Bohm, D. (1980/1983) *Wholeness and the Implicate Order*. London: ARK.

Brown, F.A. Jr., Hastings, J.W. and Palmer, J.D. (1970) *The Biological Clock*. New York: Academic Press.

Clark, P.A. (1982) *A Review of the Theories of Time and Structure for Organisational Sociology*. Birmingham: The University of Aston Management Centre, Working Paper Series.

Cloudsley-Thompson, J.L. (1980) *Biological Clocks. Their Functions in Nature*. London: Weidenfeld and Nicolson.

Conroy, R. and Mills, J.M. (1971) *Human Circadian Rhythms*. Baltimore: Williams and Wilkins.

Dirken, J.M. (1966) 'Industrial Shift Work: Decrease in Wellbeing and Specific Effects', *Ergonomics*, 9(2): 115–24.

Dossey, L. (1982) *Space, Time and Medicine*. London: Shambala.

Estrote, Sue E. (1982) *Making it Crazy: An Ethnography of Psychiatric Clients in an American Community*. Berkeley University.

Folkard, S. and Monk, T. (eds) (1985) *Hours of Work. Temporal Factors in Work Scheduling*. Chichester: Wiley.

Fraser, J.T. (1982) *The Genesis and Evolution of Time*. Brighton: Harvester Press.

Fraser, J.T. (1987) *Time the Familiar Stranger*. Amherst: University of Massachusetts Press.

Graham, H. (1990) *Time, Energy and the Psychology of Healing*. London: Jessica Kingsley.

Heimann, H. (1983) 'Zeitstrukturen in der Psychopathalogie', in A. Peisl and A. Mohler (eds), *Die Zeit*. München: R. Oldenburg. pp. 59–78.

Luce, G.G. (1973) *Body Time. The Natural Rhythms of the Body*. St Albans, Herts: Paladin.

Luhmann, N. (1982) 'World-Time and System History', in *The Differentiation of Society*. New York: Columbia University Press. pp. 289–324.

Mead, G.H. (1932/1959) *The Philosophy of the Present*, ed. by A.E. Murphy, with a Preface by John Dewey. La Salle, Ill.: Open Court.

Melbin, M. (1987) *Night as Frontier. Colonizing the World after Dark*. New York: The Free Press, Macmillan.

Melges, F.T. (1982) *Time and the Inner Future: A Temporal Approach to Psychiatric Disorders*. New York: Wiley.

Merloo, J.A.M. (1970) *Along the Fourth Dimension: Man's Sense of Time and History*. New York: John Day.

Mitford, J. (1963) *The American Way of Death*. New York: Fawcett.

Payk, T.R. (1979) *Mensch und Zeit. Chronopathologie im Grundriss*. Stuttgart: Hippokrates Verlag.

Prigogine, I. (1980) *From Being to Becoming. Time and Complexity in the Physical Sciences*. San Francisco: W.H. Freemann.

Reinberg, A. and Ghata, J. (1965) *Biological Rhythms*. New York: Walker and Son.

Reinberg, A., Ardlouer, P., De Prims, J., Malbecq, W., Vieux, N. and Bourdeleau, P. (1984) 'Desynchronisation of the Oral Temperature, Circadian Rhythm and Intolerance to Shift Work', *Nature*, 308(5956): 272–4.

Rinderspacher, J.P. (1985) *Gesellschaft ohne Zeit. Individuelle Zeitverwendung und soziale Organisation der Arbeit*. Frankfurt am Main: Campus Verlag.

Rose, K.J. (1989) *The Body in Time*. New York: Wiley.

Scheller, H. (1963) 'Korsakow-Syndrom und Zeitlichkeit', in G. Schaltenbrand (ed.), *Zeit in nervenärztlicher Sicht*. Stuttgart: Ferdinand Enke. pp. 79–87.

Thompson, E.P. (1967) 'Time, work-discipline, and industrial capitalism', *Past and Present*, 36: 57–97.

Young, M. (1988) *The Metronomic Society. Natural Rhythms and Human Timetables*. London: Thames and Hudson.

Index

and disease, distinguished, 6
and moral values, 46–51
necessity of adding concept sickness
  to, 6–7
relationship to suffering, 7
time in, 7–8
time of onset revised, 8
illth, 6, 153
infertility treatment, 60
Inuit (Arctic), 83
Italy, 12, 68–74
  and US compared 72

Jahoda, Marie, 16, 143–4
James, Allison, 123
Japanese, 38
Jaques, Eliot, 38, 41–2, 85, 117
Jenkins Activity Scale, 31
Jung, Carl, 21

Klein, Rudolph, 102
Kleinman, Arthur, 6–7
Kushlick, Albert, 10, 17

labour (childbirth),
  length of, 69
    as supposed indication of pathology,
      72
  -ward, 56
    time perceptions in, 73
    gesture speed in, 73
Lakoff and Johnson, 148–9
Law, John, 7
Leathard, Audrey, 61
Leeson, Joyce, 7
Lehmann, Rosamund, 61
Lewis, E., 64
Lewis, Gilbert, 6, 8–9, 12
Lewis, Ieuan, 12
lifecourse, 86–7
  as flowing current, 141
  as journey, 141
'lifedeath', 7
lifestyle as etiological factor, 34
'liminality', 137
'limited good', 49
Littlewood and Lipsedge, 50
Lodge, Peter, 7
Luce, G.G., 155, 156
Luhmann, Niklas, 154
Lupton, Tom, 109

Lusaka (Zambia), 12

McKenna, F., 109
Malaise Inventory, 147
manager's time, 111
Mann, Thomas, 17, 23
manual work,
  and dance, 113
Marmot, M.G., 32
Martin, Emily, 56
Marx, Karl, 8, 16, 18, 41, 112
Masai (Kenya), 27
MASH, 24
Mauss, Marcel, 21
Measor and Woods, 126
medicine,
  as delinquent community, 105
  history taking, 11, 13, 20–1
  hegemony attacked, 101
  holistic, 139
  and unemployment, 147–8
  as waiting culture, 1
Melbin, Murray, 156
menarche, 57
  timing of, 57
menstruation *see also* periods, 57–60
  diverse meanings, 59–60
  regularity of cycle, 57–8
  rescheduling, 59–60
  time transitions in, 57
  untimeliness, 60
  workplace problems, 58
mental health, 158–9
metaphors,
  fitness for promotion, 127
  general discussion, 148–9
  Hamlet's Queen, 105
  importance of making explicit, 89–90,
    91
  juggling act, 108
  knights in shining armour, 90
  maiden in distress, 90
  medical applied to GP organization, 78
  midwives, 18
  monastic orders, 21, 145
  pilgrimage, 12, 23
  railway train as General Practice, 79–80
  railways, 110
  roads, rivers, ribbons, 40
  sexual, 24
  ship at sea, 23